Account of the Native Africans in the Neighbourhood of Sierra Leone

To Which is Added, An Account of the Present State of Medicine Among Them

VOLUME 2

THOMAS WINTERBOTTOM

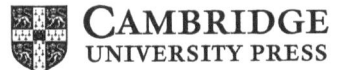

CAMBRIDGE
UNIVERSITY PRESS

CAMBRIDGE UNIVERSITY PRESS

Cambridge, New York, Melbourne, Madrid, Cape Town, Singapore,
São Paolo, Delhi, Dubai, Tokyo, Mexico City

Published in the United States of America by Cambridge University Press, New York

www.cambridge.org
Information on this title: www.cambridge.org/9781108020879

© in this compilation Cambridge University Press 2010

This edition first published 1803
This digitally printed version 2010

ISBN 978-1-108-02087-9 Paperback

CAMBRIDGE LIBRARY COLLECTION

Books of enduring scholarly value

History

The books reissued in this series include accounts of historical events and movements by eye-witnesses and contemporaries, as well as landmark studies that assembled significant source materials or developed new historiographical methods. The series includes work in social, political and military history on a wide range of periods and regions, giving modern scholars ready access to influential publications of the past.

Account of the Native Africans in the Neighbourhood of Sierra Leone

Sierra Leone in West Africa is the subject of this 1803 work by English physician Thomas Winterbottom (1766–1859). In the 1790s he spent four years there working for the Sierra Leone Company (established by abolitionists to resettle ex-slaves), and combating diseases such as malaria and scurvy. He displays none of the pejorative views of Africa or its inhabitants that some of his contemporaries expressed, but has a very positive opinion of the country. Winterbottom describes the women as beautiful and graceful, and he dismisses racial differentiations based on skin colour as being absurd. In Volume 2 Winterbottom focuses on African medicine and common diseases found in Sierra Leone. He pays particular attention to cases of abortions and miscarriages, and to malnourished children. The author does not refrain from addressing circumcision and sexually transmitted diseases, and is intrigued by the role of magic in the native medical tradition.

Cambridge University Press has long been a pioneer in the reissuing of out-of-print titles from its own backlist, producing digital reprints of books that are still sought after by scholars and students but could not be reprinted economically using traditional technology. The Cambridge Library Collection extends this activity to a wider range of books which are still of importance to researchers and professionals, either for the source material they contain, or as landmarks in the history of their academic discipline.

Drawing from the world-renowned collections in the Cambridge University Library, and guided by the advice of experts in each subject area, Cambridge University Press is using state-of-the-art scanning machines in its own Printing House to capture the content of each book selected for inclusion. The files are processed to give a consistently clear, crisp image, and the books finished to the high quality standard for which the Press is recognised around the world. The latest print-on-demand technology ensures that the books will remain available indefinitely, and that orders for single or multiple copies can quickly be supplied.

The Cambridge Library Collection will bring back to life books of enduring scholarly value (including out-of-copyright works originally issued by other publishers) across a wide range of disciplines in the humanities and social sciences and in science and technology.

AN

ACCOUNT

OF THE

NATIVE AFRICANS

IN THE NEIGHBOURHOOD OF

SIERRA LEONE;

TO WHICH IS ADDED,

AN ACCOUNT

OF THE

PRESENT STATE OF MEDICINE AMONG THEM.

Come fanciul ch'a pena
Volge la Lingua e snoda;
Che dir non sa, ma 'l più tacer gli è Noia
Così 'l desir mi mena
A dire :———
Mi palpita il cor!———ma forse diran
............,che un primo. Errore
Punir non si dovea ; che un Ramo infermo
Subito non recide saggio Cultor.

BY

THOMAS WINTERBOTTOM, M. D.

PHYSICIAN TO THE COLONY OF SIERRA LEONE.

VOL. II.

LONDON:

PRINTED BY C. WHITTINGHAM,
Dean Street ;

AND SOLD BY JOHN HATCHARD, 199, PICCADILLY,
AND J. MAWMAN, POULTRY,

1803

CONTENTS.

VOLUME II.

CHAP. I.

Page

*Introduction—Origin of Medicine—First Physicians—Union
of Medicine and Magic—Practice of Medicine in Africa—
General Division* 1

CHAP. II.

GENERAL DISEASES.

*Fever—Remedies for the Thirst, Vomiting, and Head-ach
which attend it—Remittents—Mode of Cupping—Intermittents—Enlargement of the Spleen—Œdema of lower Extremities—Mania—Idiotism—Epilepsy—Worms—Lethargy* 13

CHAP. III.

*Venereal Disease—Gonorrhœa—Phlegmone Testis—Hernia—
Coup de Soleil—Tooth-ache—Scurvy—Ear-ach—Dysen-
tery on board of Slave Ships; on Shore—Diarrhœa—
Cholic* 32

CHAP. IV.

Elephantiasis 50

CHAP. V.

Dracunculus or Guinea Worm—Chigres 82

CHAP VI.

*Enlargement of the Scrotum—Enlargement of the Legs—
Gout—Rheumatism—Pleurisy—Diseased Liver—Scrophula—Phthisis—Anorexia—Spitting of Blood* 110

CHAP. VII.

*Diseases of the Eyes—Nyctalopia—Case of Croup—Sore
Throat—Corpulency—Small Pox—Inoculation—Measles* 127

CONTENTS.

CHAP. VIII.

Yaws... 139

CHAP. IX.

Herpes—Krakra—Mottled Appearance of Skin—Effects of Fish
Poison—Nostalgia 163

CHAP X.

Bite of Snakes—Of Scorpions—Of Tarantulas 176

CHAP. XI.

Burns and Scalds—Ulcers—Recent Wounds—Fractures 193

CHAP. XII.

THE DISEASES OF WOMEN—WITH THE SEXUAL PECULIARITIES IN AFRICA.

Hysteria—Catamenia—Labours—Expulsion of the Placenta—
Abortion—Miscarriage—Milk Breasts—Pendulous Bel-
lies—Suckling... 205

CHAP. XIII.

THE DISEASES AND MANAGEMENT OF CHILDREN.

Treatment after the Birth—Locked Jaw—Method of carrying
Children—Eruptions—Indistinct Articulation—Tinea Capitis—Weakness—Wasting—Diarrhœa—Protrusions of the
Navel—Rickets—Prolapsus Ani—Dirt-eating—Large Bel-
lies 219

APPENDIX. No. I. An Account of Circumcision as it is practised on the Windward Coast of Africa 229

APPENDIX. No. II. An Account of the African Bark 243

APPENDIX. No. III. Remarks suggested by the Perusal of
Mr. White's Work on the regular Gradation in Man 254

APPENDIX. No. IV. Remarks of Professor Blumenbach
upon Negroes... 275

PRESENT STATE OF MEDICINE

AMONG

THE NATIVES

OF

SIERRA LEONE.

CHAP. I.

INTRODUCTION. ORIGIN OF MEDICINE. FIRST PHY-
SICIANS. UNION OF MEDICINE AND MAGIC. PRAC-
TICE OF MEDICINE IN AFRICA. GENERAL DIVISION.

THE following attempt to sketch a history of
the present state of medicine among the
natives of Africa, and to give some account of
those diseases to which they are more peculiarly
liable, was undertaken during the calamitous and
distressed state to which the colony of Sierra
Leone was reduced, in consequence of the depre-
dations committed there by the French, in the
year 1794. It was resorted to with the view of
restoring some degree of activity to a mind
broken down by sickness, and afflicted by the

scenes of distress which daily presented themselves. This account must unavoidably prove very defective; partly from a want of knowledge of the different languages spoken by the nations who are the subject of it, and partly from the great unwillingness which they shew to disclose the secrets of their medical art. The inconveniences which are produced by the former circumstance, are but imperfectly remedied by the assistance of an interpreter; and the difficulties which result from the latter are well pointed out by Dr. Rush, who is so deservedly eminent as a physician and philosopher, in his Inquiry into the Natural History of Medicine among the Indians of North America *. "By what arts," says he, "shall we persuade them to discover their remedies? and how shall we come at the knowledge of facts in that cloud of errors in which, the credulity of the Europeans, and the superstition of the Indians, have involved both their diseases and remedies? These difficulties serve to increase the importance of our subject. If I should not be able to solve them, perhaps I may lead the way to more successful endeavours for that purpose."

An inquiry of this kind, were the obstacles which oppose its prosecution entirely removed, would no doubt prove sufficiently interesting. We are indebted to the experience of nations, more rude than those of Africa, and inhabiting countries which possess fewer natural advantages, for some of our most valuable remedies. We have

* Medical Inquiries, vol. i.

therefore some reason to hope, that as Africa, though hitherto too much neglected, has already enriched many European arts by its productions, so it may have in store for future observers some articles which may become important acquisitions to the materia medica;

Some " herbs, and potent trees, and drops of balm,
Rich with the genial influence of the sun,
To brace the nerveless arm, with food to win
Sick appetite, or hush th' unquiet breast *."

Considerable pains have been taken to discover those remedies upon which the natives place their chief dependance for the cure of diseases; and to prevent, as much as possible, any ambiguity arising in default of scientific names, as many of the native names of vegetables, &c. as could be procured, have been inserted. For the Linnæan names of medical plants which have been mentioned, I am indebted to my learned friend Dr. Adam Afzelius, demonstrator of botany in the university of Upsala, who has kindly promised to supply such as are wanting, in the elaborate work which he is now preparing on the natural history of Sierra Leone.

Although the present account relates chiefly to the Timmanees and Bulloms, who inhabit the banks of the Sierra Leone and its neighbourhood, yet the customs of other nations, particularly those dwelling to the northward of that river, will be occasionally noticed, where an opportunity has occurred of observing any striking

* Akenside.

differences between them. Indeed it is highly probable that the same medical customs will be found to prevail, more or less, for several hundred miles along the coast of Africa, as a very great similarity of manners prevails among the inhabitants, although divided into so many different nations.

The origin of medicine has probably been the same in every country, and its progress towards perfection has been equally slow and gradual in all. To relieve the body from sickness and pain must early have excited the attention of mankind. The rudest nations we are acquainted with have a knowledge of medicine. Pliny observes, that if at any time there have been people without physicians, yet they have not been without medicines; and the science remained at Rome, even after the physicians had been banished from the city. It is in the savage state, or the state of nature as it is called, that that part of medicine which attends chiefly to accidents is more peculiarly requisite *; for men, whilst engaged in hunting wild beasts, or while roaming over an uncultivated country, covered with impenetrable forests, are more exposed to wounds, bruises, and other accidents, than those who live in a more civilized state; hence it is probable that some degree of medical experience must have been coeval with the origin of mankind. Quintilian

* Medicina quondam paucarum fuit scientia herbarum, quibus sisteretur fluens sanguis, vulnera coirent paulatim. Seneca Epistol. 95.

remarks, " Medicina ex observatione salubrium atque his contrariorum reperta est ; et ut quibusdam placet, tota constat experimentis. Nam et vulnus deligavit aliquis antequam hæc ars esset : et febrem quiete et abstinentia, non quia rationem videbat, sed quia id valetudo ipsa coegerat, mitigavit *."

As it is more obscure in its nature than other. arts, so medicine has been slower in its progress. In some instances we are said to have been indebted to the practice of animals for the knowledge of particular remedies; in other instances to accident, or to a fancied resemblance between a plant and the disease it was supposed to cure †. Even at this time many medicines are retained in the materia medica of European nations from some such fanciful notion of their virtues. Among the many histories of accidental discoveries of

* Institut. II. xviii.

† Pliny says " Hippopotamus in quadam medendi parte etiam *magister* exstitit. Assidua namque satietate obesus, exit in litus, recentes arundinum cæsuras speculatum: atque ubi acutissimum videt stirpem, imprimens corpus, venam quandam in crure vulnerat, atque ita profluvio sanguinis morbidum alias corpus exonerat, et plagam limo rursus obducit.

Simile quiddam et volucris in eadem Ægypto monstravit, quæ vocatur ibis: rostri aduncitate per eam partem se perluens, qua reddi ciborum onera maxime salubre est. Nec hæc sola a multis animalibus reperta sunt, usui futura et homini ; for which consult Pliny Lib. viii. c. 27.

In another place he observes, " Torpescunt scorpiones aconiti tactu—Auxiliatur his elleborum album—Tangunt carnes aconito, necantque gustatu earum pantheras :—at illas statim liberari morte, excrementorum hominis gustu, demonstratum.—Pudendumque rursus, omnia animalia, quæ sint salutaria ipsis, nosse, præter hominem." L. xxvii. c 2.

remedies, that of the purgative effects of helle-
bore by Melampus bears at least an air of probability, as also does that of the Peruvian bark.

From history we learn, that the practice of medicine formed a part of the duties of religion among
the chief nations of antiquity ; perhaps from this
consideration, that the priests of the gods were
alone thought worthy to practise an art so much
beyond the reach of human genius to discover,
and of which they boasted that the gods themselves were the inventors. Kings were formerly
instructed in this art, and philosophers considered
medicine as one of the chief objects of their attention ; among others, Aristotle is said to have practised medicine before he applied to the study of
philosophy.

The first account we have of physicians is contained in the sacred writers, where they are also
said to be embalmers of the dead. The " art of
the apothecary is also frequently noticed ; but
though they might occasionally have practised
physic, they appear to have been chiefly venders
of drugs, myropolæ ; and afterwards, when physic
became a distinct branch of science, this art fell
into contempt, and probably became that of a
mere perfumer, unguentarius *.

At the same time quackery may have drawn
its origin : a kind of gypsies or fortune-tellers,
called by the antients agyrtæ, æruscatores †,
præstigiatores, &c. pretended to cure diseases by

---

* Cic. Offic. i. 42.   † Calepin Dict. und. Ling.

charms, and by a variety of mysterious ceremonies. These people also, like the greegree men in Africa, or the obia professors in the West Indies, wreaked their vengeance upon those who offended them, by the recital of magic verses. " Irritat, mulcet, falsis terroribus implet."

In all the uncultivated nations of antiquity, medicine has been held in the highest esteem, and even considered as a divine art. Homer often speaks of the peculiar respect paid to those who were skilled to dress a

> Wound with drugs of pain assuaging power;

an art which had not been neglected by the haughty * Achilles.

Medicine, as well as many other useful arts, appears to have been very early cultivated in Egypt, as is evident in the sacred writings. *Homer* calls Egypt the land of physicians, and says,

> ————Egypt teems with drugs, yielding no few,
> Which, mingled with the drink, are good, and many
> Of baneful juice, and enemies to life.
> There ev'ry man in skill medicinal
> Excels, for they are sons of Pæon all †.

Pliny also says, medicinam Ægyptii apud ipsos volunt repertam : alii per Arabum, Babylonis et Apollinis filium : herbariam et medicamentariam a Chirone ; hence it appears that we are indebted,

---

* See the story of Democedes, related by Herodotus, iii. 129; also Ecclesiasticus, ch. xxxviii.

† Odyss. iv. 288, by Cowper.

for at least the rudiments of this art, to the Africans, despicable as their knowledge of it may appear to us at present.

This union of medicine with the ceremonies of religion, which occurred during the early ages of mankind, among all those nations of whom we have any records, is also found to prevail amongst all those with whom navigation has lately made us acquainted; and both appear to have been universally connected with those superstitious practices, the magicæ vanitates, which from time immemorial have kept the minds of mankind in a constant state of alarm. Pliny, speaking of this triple union, says of magic in particular, " Natam primam e medicina nemo dubitat, ac specie salutari irrepsisse velut altiorem sanctioremque medicinam : ita blandissimis desideratissimisque promissis addidisse vires religionis, ad quas maxime etiamnum caligat humanum genus *." The dependency of medicine upon magic, or at least upon the same disposition of mind, is not yet broken, and if formerly they " with incantation staunch'd the sable blood," the same natural effect is frequently, at the present day, attributed to causes equally trifling and ridiculous. The Druids were priests and physicians among the Gauls and ancient Britains. In North America, the priests of the Indians are at the same time their physicians and their conjurors ; whilst they heal their wounds, or cure their diseases, they interpret their dreams, give them protective charms, and satisfy that de-

* Lib. xxxi. c. 1.

sire which is so prevalent among them of search-
ing into futurity *. It is curious to remark, that
the same notion respecting medicine prevails
among the islanders of the South Seas. At Otaheite, a physician is called tahauwamai, a word
compounded of tahauwa, a priest, and mai, pain.
Thus we see that all nations, while in similar
states of cultivation, possess nearly the same ideas,
though cut off from all communication by immense tracts of ocean.

Respecting the practice of medicine in Africa,
there is reason to imagine that it is not at present in a progressive state of improvement, but
that it remains nearly as it was some centuries
ago. This arises chiefly from their great repug-
nance to change customs which long usage has
rendered venerable. They plant their rice, build
their houses, and manufacture their cloth in exactly the same manner as their forefathers, and
they answer every objection, by saying it is
" country fashion." This attachment, however,
to long established customs, though probably
strengthened in tropical climates by the enervat-
ing power of heat, is not peculiar to the Africans:
it is observed to prevail in all countries parti-
ally civilized. Thus the manners and customs
of the Asiatics, as described in scripture, are nearly
the same as those which are observed in the East
at the present day †.

* Carver's Travels in North America.
† Spirit of Laws, xiv. 4.

The notions respecting the effects of medicine are, in Africa, so much blended with a regard to magical ceremonies and incantations, that it is often difficult to discover on which they chiefly rely for success. Although they imagine that every disease attended with danger is occasioned by witchcraft or poison *, yet they readily admit that sickness may occur independently of these causes. In support of this opinion they argue, that if a vessel of any kind be filled with clean water every day, and be not washed out, it must at length become foul; hence, say they, arises the necessity of washing the stomach from time to time with some medicine, although unattended with any operative effects. Another reason why they suppose the stomach to be the chief seat of disease, is the loss of appetite, which so frequently attends it, and which is to them the most alarming symptom. When the body is disordered, from whatever cause, they do not believe that it can be again restored to health simply by its own powers, or by the powers of nature as they are called, of which they have not the smallest notion.

In collecting medicines for use, they pay no regard to the phases of the moon, nor do they refer any of their diseases to the influence of this

---

* The Bulloms have a saying among them, that a Bullom man cannot die unless his death be occasioned by poison or witchcraft. Van Helmont appears to have entertained the same notion, when he says, Deus non fecit mortem.
DE LITHIASI, C. V.

planet. Those who live upon the coast are of opinion, that people can only die at high or low tide. The influence of the tide upon departing life has long been credited ; Piso says, during the six hours of the increase of the tide, diseases are exacerbated and pains are greatly increased ; but that they gradually abate during the reflux. The same author appears firmly persuaded that men die only during the ebb tide. Dr. Haller supposes that Piso was the first who formed this opinion; but Aristotle fell into the same error, and asserts that no animal dies during the increase of the tide *.

It is very common for those who are indisposed, to go and reside for some time in a distant village †, in order to take medicines from some one who has acquired celebrity for the cure of a particular disorder ; this is frequently some old woman, to whom even Europeans will often trust themselves in preference to their own countrymen ‡.

* Haller Bib. Med. Pract. iii. 1.
† Jeremiah xlvi. 11.
‡ Atkins gives an instance of this adherence to the superstitious practices of the natives, in a governor of Cape Coast Castle, General Phips. " The general," he observes, " has taken a *consa*, which by the negroes is understood a temporary wife ; she is a mulatto-woman, begot by a Dutch soldier at des Minas, by whom he has four children, of *fair flaxen hair* and *complexion*. He dotes on this woman, whom he persuades now and then to our chapel service, and she complies without devotion, being a strict adherer to the *negrish* customs. I attended the illness of one of her children, and afterwards on the General himself, who, on both occasions, I found, was so weak or so wise, as to give the preference of *fetishing* to any physical directions of mine,

In prosecuting the inquiry into the diseases of the Africans, I shall consider,

1. General diseases, to which both sexes are liable.

2. The diseases of women, with the sexual peculiarities in Africa.

3. The diseases and management of children.

---

wearing them on his wrists and neck. He was a gentleman of good sense, yet could not help yielding to the silly customs created by our fears." Having given this instance of the governor's weakness, it may not be improper to notice what this writer further adds on this subject, which may serve as a proof of the good understanding of his lady. " He cannot persuade this woman to leave the country, though he has stole or forced her consent for all the children, in regard to their education ; she still conforming to the dress of her country, being always barefoot and fetished with chains and gobbets of gold, at her ancles, her wrists, and her hair; to alter which in England, *she thinks, would sit awkward, and, together with her ignorance how to comport herself with new and strange conversation, would, in all likelihood alienate her husband's affections.*"

CHAP. II.

GENERAL DISEASES.

FEVER. REMEDIES FOR THE THIRST, VOMITING, AND HEADACH, WHICH ATTEND IT. REMITTENTS. MODE OF CUPPING. INTERMITTENTS. ENLARGEMENT OF THE SPLEEN. ŒDEMA OF LOWER EXTREMITIES. MANIA. IDIOTISM. EPILEPSY. WORMS. LE- THARGY.

FEVER is the most frequent and most fatal disease to which Europeans are subject upon this coast : it is less common among the Africans, who also suffer less from its attacks. In them, it is generally the sequel of a debauch, and very frequently follows the excessive intemperance in which they indulge at the funeral of their friends. It is a common remark among them, that one ' *cry*' is generally followed by several others ; for when any person of consequence dies, several others fall sick, and often narrowly escape with their lives. Even this they attribute to witch-craft, though it evidently depends upon their own misconduct. They have no idea of the nature of fever, as a general disease, nor have they any word in their language to express it, but name it from any of its urgent symptoms, as *sick head**, *sick belly*, &c. On that account it has been supposed that the Africans are not liable to the attacks of remittent fever, an opinion which is contrary to fact. It is not

* Head-ach in Bullom is, Bul nek-kée-ay ; in Timmanee, Ro-búmp robáng. Sick belly, in Bullom, is Koonay nekkeeay ; in Timmanee, Koor Rob-báng.

uncommon to see the natives affected with slight, but distinctly formed paroxysms of fever, which sometimes terminate within twenty-four hours, and are considered as common head-achs. I have known instances where repeated paroxysms have occurred, and where the remittent fever has run its course precisely as it would have done in any European who had resided long upon the coast, and who by undergoing the *seasoning*, as it is termed, had assimilated himself to the climate. It may not be improper here to remark, that what is termed *seasoning* among Europeans, an idea peculiar to themselves, implies merely the first severe fit of illness, chiefly fever, which a person suffers after his arrival in a tropical climate; succeeding attacks of fever are usually experienced in a slighter degree, though in this respect there is great difference, for some have repeated attacks as severe as the first. Those Europeans at Sierra Leone, who longest resisted the power of climate in producing sickness, suffered more, and were more dangerously affected, than those who sickened soon after their arrival. People of fair complexions appeared to be more liable to fever, and to suffer relapses from slighter causes, than those of darker complexions, but they experienced, upon the whole, less severe attacks than the latter. From a few instances it appeared that the climate was more inimical to men above forty-five, than to those who were younger. Women enjoyed a tolerable state of health, nearly as good as in Europe; their complaints were in general less severe than those of the men, but the state of convalescence was slower, and they were more liable to be harassed with symptoms of irritability or of erethism*.

Dr. Clark, of Dominica, speaking of the yellow fever which prevailed in that island in the years 1793, 4, 5, and 6, observes, " the new negroes, who had been lately imported from the coast of Africa, were all attacked with it. The negroes who had been long in the town, or on the island, escaped."

Another accurate observer, Dr. Chisholme, of Grenada, remarks, that, " although it is probable that the negro race possess something constitutional, which resists the action of contagion in a very great degree, still it must be admitted that their necessary temperance must have contributed much in the present instance to their exemption from, or to the mildness of, the disease when it appeared among them." The effects of temperance, as a prophylactic, are strikingly demonstrated by the same author: " Whilst the pestilential fever raged here," he observes, " the utility of these means was remarkably illustrated by the almost total exemption of the French inhabitants from the disease. Their mode of living, compared to that of the English, is temperate and regular in an uncommon degree†."

* Vide Med. Facts, vol. viii.

† Dr. Chisholme, in the work quoted above, entitled, " An Essay on the malignant pestilential Fever introduced into the West Indian Islands, from Bullom, on the Coast of Guinea," endeavours to prove that the disease was of African origin. But notwithstanding the instances adduced by Dr. Chisholme, of several persons who were seized with a dangerous fever soon after they had visited a vessel called the Hankey, which arrrived at Grenada

When the thirst is very distressing in fever, the pith of a species of reed called cattop, (Timmanee) sinkwonnyee or kaymanghee, (Soosoo) wishá, (Bullom) is bruised, and after being boiled for a

from the island of Bulama or Boullam ; and notwithstanding the sickly state in which this vessel is said to have been on leaving Bulama, and during the passage to the West Indies, yet there is reason to suspect that the disease in question, if really imported into those islands, did not originate from the island of Bulam. In other instances we find every specific contagion produces a disease *sui generis*, differing only in greater or less degree of violence, or at most possessing such slight deviations as are occasioned by particular states of the atmosphere, or peculiar modes of living. But in the instance of the pestilential fever described by Dr. Chisholme, we should be induced to suppose that the contagion had not merely acquired a greater degree of virulence, but had been converted into a different species.

The fever, which carried off so many of the settlers at Bulama, precisely resembled the endemial remittent fever of Sierra Leone, a sketch of which, at some future opportunity, may perhaps be laid before the public ; but the fever described by Dr. Chisholme differs so essentially from that which occurred at Sierra Leone, that it cannot be recognised as the same disease. Besides, about the same period, a fever similar to that of Grenada showed itself in the other West India Islands, and in America, particularly at Philadelphia, where no rational cause could be assigned for its appearance, which would not have been the case had it been imported.

Dr. Chisholme has committed an error, of not much consequence, indeed, in supposing that the Hankey and another ship, the Calypso, were chartered by the Sierra Leone Company (page 83) ; and further, (in page 86) he adds, " Capt. Coxe (of the Hankey) finding the water at Bullam unwholesome, proceeded with his ship to Bissao, where there is a Portuguese settlement, for a supply. The ship was navigated by about twelve seamen, most of whom had not experienced sickness, and had been probably procured from Sierra Leone." The Hankey had no communication whatever with Sierra Leone, nor do I believe she ever had a person on board from that place. The other vessel, the Calypso, after leaving Bulam, called for refreshment at Sierra Leone, where she remained about six weeks, during which time upwards of forty of the crew and passengers died of the remittent fever, though unattended with any appearance of peculiar malignity.

little time in water, the decoction is used as the common drink; it is very acid, and is very effectual in quenching thirst. They employ, for the same purpose, the delicious fruit of the ananas; which clears the mouth from sordes, and makes the tongue and gums as red, as if the blood were ready to burst forth.

Vomiting is one of the most distressing symptoms which occur in fevers: to alleviate or remove it, they drink a warm infusion of the common red pepper, or capsicum, or they swallow a few pods of it gently bruised. The juice of the lime is also frequently taken with the same intention, or they use the expressed juice of the medulla, or scraped stem of the cattop, to which is sometimes added a decoction of the leaves of a tree called by the Bulloms and Timmanees yúffo.

Head-ach is another symptom of fever which frequently causes much uneasiness and distress to the patient, and, on that account, cephalics form a most numerous class of remedies in the African materia medica: in fact, there are but.few plants, particularly such as possess a degree of aroma, which they do not suppose to be good for the head. Almost the whole of these remedies are applied externally, chiefly to the forehead; the only thing used internally being an infusion of the scoparia dulcis, which is sometimes drunk warm like tea. The most celebrated of their external applications are the following. 1. Abúnk (Timmanee). The leaves are bruised between two stones, and formed into a kind of paste with water, which is rubbed upon the forehead twice a day, and repeated for at least a week.

2. The leaves of a plant called cooteè (Timmanee) are bruised and made into a paste with water, and applied in the same manner as abunk. This herb has a very delightful odour, resembling that of the anthoxanthum odoratum, which imparts the fragrance to new mown hay, and is used by the natives to smell at.

3. The leaves of the lime bush, when beaten in a mortar, are afterwards heated in an iron pot and applied hot, wrapped in a handkerchief, to the forehead; they are much commended for their efficacy in this complaint.

4. A remedy, the reverse to the above, consists in applying the cold leaves of the plantain tree to the forehead, which are renewed as often as they grow warm. The grateful coolness of these leaves frequently produces a temporary abatement of the excruciating pain which attends the exacerbation of their fevers*.

5. Comamboy (Timmanee), mamboy (Bullom). The seed, which is as large as a chesnut, is finely scraped, and rubbed over the forehead : as it is of a very hot and acrid nature, if it be too long applied, it produces nearly the same effects as cantharides.

* Professor Thunberg, speaking of the ricinus, says, " the leaves of the shrub dried, and applied round the head, were affirmed to be serviceable in the head-ach," probably from their coolness.

6. Apúntokellee (Timmanee), Issumpellén (Bullom), Santáy (Soosoo), mimosa involuta*. The whole of the leaves and smaller branches are bruised, and applied cold to the forehead, as a poultice. A decoction of it is also frequently used to bathe the face and gums when painful and swoln.

7. Mabúnk (Timmanee). The dried leaves of this plant are powdered, and applied to the forehead, softened with water.

8. Matakkee (Timmanee). This is used in the same manner as the above; it is a hot, acrid plant, and is frequently applied to the head to kill vermin.

9. Abák (Timmanee). The dry leaves are powdered, and used like those of matakkee.

10. Manai (Timmanee). The fresh panicles of the plant are rubbed over the forehead.

11. Mattopper (Timmanee). This is a warm, aromatic odorous plant, having a strong, bitter taste : the leaves are applied to the forehead as in the preceding instances. The red berries of this tree somewhat resemble cherries, and are eagerly sought after by a species of dove with a bright green plumage.

12. Tunkámúntoo (Timmanee). The leaves are boiled in water, and used warm for washing the forehead.

---

* The bark of this tree is used to make a coarse kind of mat.

† The bark of mattopper is used by the natives to dye leather of a red colour. The bark is beaten small, and infused in water gently heated, and the leather is suffered to remain a few hours in the mixture.

13. Mapóor (Timmanee). A species of af-
zelia. The leaves dried in the sun are powdered,
and mixed with water so as to form a cataplasm,
and applied cold to the forehead.

14. The leaves of a plant, called by the Soosoos
makóotay, are applied in the same manner as
those of mapóor.

15. Agbunto (Timmanee). This is a very
warm aromatic plant, resembling thyme in taste.
An infusion of the whole plant is drank warm for
the purpose of producing perspiration, and at the
same time the leaves are rubbed upon the forehead. A decoction of the leaves of the two
following plants are used solely for bathing the
forehead.

16. Quéequee or Maquéequee (Timmanee).

17. Teechee (Timmanee).

18. Teebooraкee (Timmanee), is a plant used
for the cure of head-ach when accompanied with
sore throat; it has an aromatic taste, and resembles sage in smell, and appears to be chiefly used
as a sudorific.

When the head-ach proves obstinate, and does
not yield to these means, they have recourse to
cupping, which is the only method of drawing
blood they are acquainted with. Prosper Alpinus
asserts, that the Egyptians used to draw blood
from both the arteries and veins, a practice unknown upon the western coast of this continent.
Cupping is generally performed by some old woman; who makes first a number of small incisions, with a sharp pointed knife, in the skin,

upon the temples or forehead, as near as possible to the seat of the pain. She then places over the incisions a cup, formed of a small gourd cut in two, the air being first rarefied by burning a little dry grass or cotton in it.

It is a custom with some, when affected with head-ach, to lie upon the hearth before a large fire, having a heavy stone laid upon one side of the head. A similar practice seems to be followed by the Mongearts, a nation of Africa, who " in head-ach bind the head with such extraordinary violence as to force out the blood from the forehead *."

Intermittents are very uncommon among the Bulloms and Timmanees, many of them having never seen the disease, except perhaps among Europeans. Hence they have no specific name for an ague, but generally term it the " shaking sickness." In the Foola country, intermittents are more usual than in the Soosoo or Mandingo countries, and they are said to be rather frequent at Teembo during the rainy season. The Mandingos and Foolas call this disease gondeea, and the Soosoos term it foorakee. When it occurs, their mode of cure consists in exciting a profuse perspiration; this is done by causing the patient to sit over a large pot in which some leaves have been boiled, the steam being confined by a large cotton cloth thrown over the patient's head, and reaching to the ground. Among the

* Saugnier and Brisson's Voyages to the Coast of Africa.

Soosoos it is usual to boil the leaves of a species
of bean tree called killéeng, previously bruised,
with which the body is bathed as a cure for this
disease.

Aguish complaints are equally uncommon
among the negro slaves in the West India Islands.
Dr. Curten, physician at Rio Bueno, Jamaica,
speaking of the negroes, says, " I have not met
among them with a pure tertian intermittent in
the whole of my practice, though white people
are often affected with them. I have been informed by practitioners of forty years experience,
that it is a rare occurrence among negroes; that
they have not met with more than one or two
instances in the whole of their practice; and
that even these few have been confined to mulattoes and house negroes, or those who live in
the same manner as white people*." The Nova
Scotian blacks settled at Free Town are, however,
very liable to agues: the only difference between
them and Europeans in this respect is, that the
former appear to suffer less from the disease, and
that in the remittent fever, the remissions are more
perfect among the Nova Scotians, and more disposed to assume the form of an intermittent.

The Africans are very seldom affected with enlargements of the spleen, or *ague cakes*, as they
are called in the fenny counties of England. They
arise from the frequent repetition of intermitting
fevers, and prove fatal to Europeans, by laying

* Ed. Med. Com. Vol. V. Dec. II.

the foundation of dropsy, and other diseases. Dr. Isert observes, that, " a negro will scarce ever be found troubled with this complaint, though almost half the Europeans on the coast have it, or at least think they have it*."

* The tumefied bellies, with which Europeans are sometimes affected in Africa, arise chiefly from enlargements of the spleen, which admits of extension to an immense bulk. In some instances it reaches as low as the crista of the ilium, and projects considerably into the right side of the abdomen. The chief uneasiness which it excites in the patient, whilst its bulk continues moderate, is a sense of weight scarcely noticed, but generally increased by lying on the right side. In process of time, when intemperance joined with repeated attacks of fever, which are permitted to run their course, have increased its bulk considerably, dyspeptic symptoms are added, in consequence of the pressure on the stomach. The liver also, though untainted with disease, suffers in its turn, chiefly from the mechanical obstruction it receives from the spleen, and partly from its connection with the stomach. Hence arises that dirty, yellow tinge, so visible in the countenances of Europeans who have resided long in Africa. Symptoms of irritation occasionally harass the patient, and are always attributed to the tumor; but seem to be less connected with it than with some recent debauch. Enlarged spleens are frequently met with in children, in whom they seldom occasion much inconvenience, but, in process of time, either totally disappear, or become so much smaller as not to attract notice. The only medicine which I have found serviceable in this complaint, is the sal cathart. given in proper doses to keep the bowels moderately open : bitter tonics were also of use in strengthening the constitution and diminishing its irritability. Mercury has little effect in reducing these tumors, and such is the irritability of the system, that even small doses are apt to affect the mouth speedily, and distress the patient greatly. Enlargements of the spleen have been referred, by those who are prejudiced against it, to the use of Peruvian bark in febrile complaints; on the contrary, they afford the strongest testimony in support of the efficacy of that invaluable medicine. Among the numerous instances of remittent and intermittent fevers, at Free Town, which were cured by a liberal use of the bark, there did not occur, at *any period*, a single

Œdematous swellings of the lower extremities, in consequence of the debility induced by frequent repetitions of the remittent and intermittent fevers, are not unfrequent complaints about Sierra Leone. They are also said to be frequent upon the Coast of Angola, and to prove soon fatal: upon the Windward Coast they generally succeed the remittent fever, but further south they are more usually the consequence of fluxes. For the cure, they heat in an iron pot a quantity of the leaves of a tree called by the Bulloms dee or lay, by the Timmanees malip, and by the Soosoos lóogree; when sufficiently warm, the leaves are applied to the leg, which is rubbed at the same time downwards with some degree of force. A decoction of the same leaf in water is often used warm as a fomentation, or bath, for the legs. The leaf of the malip has a slightly acid, astringent taste.

The castor nut, ricinus, is likewise much recommended for anasarcous swellings: the leaves, which are very mucilaginous, are steeped in hot water, and then wrapped round the leg as warm as the patient can bear, and repeated before they lose their heat. After the leaves have been thus applied for a quarter or half an hour, the limb is well dried, and the patient is put to bed, where a copious perspiration of the part generally ensues. Together with the above methods, active purgatives are occasionally used.

instance of visceral obstructions; these always arose from *neglected* attacks of fever, in which the bark had been totally omitted, or exhibited irregularly and in insufficient quantities.

The tóma, or poison tree, though so much dreaded when taken internally, is greatly celebrated as an external application in dropsical swellings of the limbs: the bark of the tree is powdered, and moistened with cold water, so as to form a cataplasm, which is said to cause the water to exude from the limb, and speedily to remove the disease, though it does not appear to be possessed of any caustic quality.

The leaves of comamboy (Timmanee), mamboy (Bullom), are beaten in a mortar, and applied cold to the legs in œdema. Care must be taken not to continue them too long, lest the part be blistered.

Persons who have fallen into a bad state of health without any evident cause, or who are convalescent from fever, &c. but still continue weak and debilitated, are washed very early every morning with a decoction of the leaves of these three plants, called goguoy, bombóy, wúrraree: this is always applied cold.

Mania is a disease which very rarely, if ever, occurs among them, nor could I make them comprehend the meaning of the term; the only idea they can form of it is, when they " lose their head," as they term it, in the delirium of drunkenness.

Idiotism is not a common disease, though I have seen two or three instances of it, one of which appeared to have arisen in consequence of repeated attacks of epilepsy.

An instance of epilepsy occurred to me in a man about forty years of age, remarkably robust and fleshy, who had been affected with it from childhood. His faculties did not appear to have suffered from these attacks, and he said he knew many who were affected with the same disease. The Soosoos call this complaint kooleekóolee; the Foolas, kreekreesá; the Mandingos, téeree; and the Timmanees, catóok; they do not attribute it to any particular cause, and consider it as incurable.

Worms of the intestines are well known among the Africans, and considered as a very frequent cause of diseases, particularly in children. The Timmanees and Bulloms do not distinguish the different species of worms by particular names, but use the word abilloo, worms, or abilloo rokóor, " worm sickness," to denote the whole. Among the Foolas and Mandingos, the various kinds are very accurately distinguished; the ascarides, or maw worms, are called by the Soosoos, koolee; by the Foolas, toomboo; and by the Mandingos, nyaallee. The lumbrici, or long worms, are called by the Foolas and Soosoos, tónnangho, and by the Mandingos, shoóndee. The Foolas name the tænia or tape worm, neagoómee; the Mandingos and Soosoos call it cálligbày.

The Foolas are peculiarly subject to the tape worm : this they attribute to their living so much upon milk, which, as it is very plentiful among them, constitutes a large portion of their diet. Dr. Sparman says, in the country round the Cape of Good Hope, the inhabitants are much troubled with worms, especially with the tape worm. He does not undertake to determine what may be the cause, but thinks it probable that a milk diet contributes somewhat.

The slaves, who are brought down to the *water side* by the Foolas for sale, are always infested with the tape worm; this probably arises from the very scanty and wretched diet with which they are fed in the *path*, as they term the journey, and which, from the distance they are brought inland, often lasts for many weeks, at the same time that their strength is further reduced by the heavy loads they are obliged to carry. Dr. Hasselquist says, that the lower classes of the inhabitants of Grand Cairo are very subject to the tape worm, which he attributes to their very poor diet : the Turks, who live better, are much less affected with this disease.

The Foolas are of opinion that people who drink rum are never troubled with the tape worm, and when they come down to the sea side among Europeans, those who are affected with tape worms sometimes venture to ask for this herculean remedy. Indeed, so high an opinion do they entertain of the medical virtues of this liquor, probably because they are so strictly forbidden its use, that they imagine it enters into the composition of every medicine made use of by Europeans; in consequence of which, when labouring under any very serious sickness, they prudently decline asking any questions respecting the composition of the medicines administered unto them. Some of the Mahommedans suppose that worms were originally produced by the " devil spitting upon Adam's belly." They have a number of remedies for the cure of worms, which are chiefly of a purgative quality: the following are those most generally used.

1. Tóngbee, (Timmanee); téngbee, (Bullom); tchaóokee, (Foola). A decoction of the leaves of this plant is taken every morning as a vermifuge; it produces no sensible effects, but the patient is directed to avoid drinking cold water after it.

2. Serigbailee, (Soosoo); leligunt, (Timmanee); Connarus africanus. Four or five kernels of the seeds are powdered, and taken for one dose, every morning, mixed with boiled rice. They produce no purgative effects.

3. The young leaves of a plant, called by the Timmanees kanónter, are bruised, and mixed with rice or fish. This medicine is particularly recommended against the lumbrici: it is said to be a very effectual remedy, though unattended with any sensible operation. The dry or fresh leaves are used indifferently.

4. The bark of a tree called by the Timmanees, argól, and by the Bulloms, coóntang, is beaten to a fine powder and boiled with a small quantity of the piper ethiopicum. A little of this decoction is taken every morning mixed with rice, and proves gently purgative; this is a very celebrated vermifuge. Where this medicine cannot

be given, as to children, on account of its nauseous taste, or where the stomach cannot retain it, a strong decoction of the same is used as a wash to the belly every day. In enlargements of the abdomen in children, also, when suspected to originate from worms, the bark of argol is reduced to a fine powder, and applied externally as a cataplasm. The seeds of the fruit of the papaw tree, taken internally, are said to be useful against worms.

The Africans are very subject to a species of lethargy, which they are much afraid of, as it proves fatal in every instance. The Timmanees call it márree, or, 'nluoi, and the Bulloms, nagónlôe, or kadeera: it is called by the Soosoos, kee kóllee kondee, or sleepy sickness, and by the Mandingos, seenoyúncaree, a word of similar import. This disease is very frequent in the Foola country, and it is said to be much more common in the interior parts of the country than upon the sea coast. Children are very rarely, or never, affected with this complaint, nor is it more common among slaves than among free people, though it is asserted that the slaves from Benin are very subject to it. At the commencement of the disease, the patient has commonly a ravenous appetite, eating twice the quantity of food he was accustomed to take when in health, and becoming very fat. When the disease has continued some time, the appetite declines, and the patient gradually wastes away.

Squinting occurs sometimes, though very seldom, in this disease, and in some rare instances the patient is carried off in convulsions. Small glandular tumors are sometimes observed in the neck a little before the commencement of this complaint, though probably depending rather upon accidental circumstances than upon the disease itself. Slave traders, however, appear to consider these tumors as a symptom indicating a disposition to lethargy, and they either never buy such slaves, or get quit of them as soon as they observe any such appearances. The disposition to sleep is so strong, as scarcely to leave a sufficient respite for the taking of food; even the repeated application of a whip, a remedy which has been frequently used, is hardly sufficient to keep the poor wretch awake. The repeated application of blisters and of setons has been employed by European surgeons without avail, as the disease, under every mode of treatment, usually proves fatal within three or four months. The natives are totally at a loss to what cause this complaint ought to be attributed; sweating is the only means they make use of, or from which they hope for any success: this is never tried but in incipient cases, for when the disease has been of any continuance they think it in vain to make the attempt. The root of a grass, called by the Soosoos kallee, and the dried leaves of a plant, called in Soosoo fingka, are boiled for some time in water, in an iron pot; when this is removed from the fire, the patient is seated over it, and is covered over with cotton cloths, a process which never fails to excite a copious perspiration. This mode of cure is repeated two or three times a day, and is persisted in for a considerable length of time, until the disease be carried off, or appears to be gaining ground. No internal medicines are given in the complaint.

CHAP. III.

GENERAL DISEASES.

VENEREAL DISEASE, GONORRHŒA, PHLEGMONE TESTIS.
HERNIA. COUP DE SOLEIL. TOOTH-ACH. SCURVY.
EAR-ACH. DYSENTERY, ON BOARD OF SLAVE SHIPS,
AND ON SHORE. DIARRHŒA. COLIC.

THE venereal disease is frequently met with among the natives, though there is great reason to believe that in every instance it had been first communicated by Europeans. The African physicians boast that they are able to cure this disease in all its forms, and in every stage, for which purpose they employ a variety of remedies, chiefly sudorifics or violent purgatives. It is said that they possess a plant, which, when chewed and swallowed, produces the same effects upon the constitution as mercury, exciting salivation, loosening the teeth, and causing a fœtor of the breath. The Sumatrans are said to possess a similar specific, and to cure this disease " with the decoction of a China root, called by them gadoong, which causes a salivation*." In the present instance† the medical skill of the Africans has met

---

* Marsden's History of Sumatra.

† Dr. Chisholm, enumerating the medical plants of Grenada, observes "the venereal virus has its antidotes; among these may be mentioned euphorbia tithymaloides, the mal nommé of the

with more applause than it deserves, as I am convinced that they are not acquainted with any vegetable which possesses properties resembling mercury, and when they excite a salivation, which they do in every case of syphilis, it is only by means of mercury procured from Europeans. Dr. Rush appears to entertain a similar opinion respecting the insufficiency of many of these boasted remedies. Speaking of the venereal disease among the Indians of North America, he says, that he doubts much of the efficacy of some Indian remedies for this disease, as the lobelia, ceanothus, and ranunculus, spoken of by Professor Kalm. He has been informed, he adds, that their chief remedy is a decoction of the pine tree used plentifully, and that several of them die in this disease.

The Foolas and Mandingos have a disease which they call LAANDA, of a very infectious nature, and which bears a striking resemblance to the venereal disease, though they consider them as essentially different. The laanda makes its appearance upon the glans or prepuce like a common chancre, but daily spreads, and in time destroys the whole of the penis. Dangerous hæmorrhages frequently arise in consequence of erosion, and the disease sometimes affects the throat, destroying the bones of the nose and palate.

French ; that singular plant saururus cernuus, the herbe à colet of the French ; lobelia syphilitica ; and costus spicatus, a new species[1]." It is to be regretted, the ingenious author does not mention either the mode of action of these plants, or the stages of the disease in which they are employed.

[1] History of the malignant fever of the West Indies.

Gonorrhœa is the most usual form of the venereal disease which occurs upon this coast, and it appears to be rather more frequent among the Soosoos and Mandingos, than among the Bulloms and Timmanees. They very unfortunately entertain an erroneous and cruel opinion, which prevails among the lower classes in Europe, that having connection with an healthy woman frees the infected person from the disease.

The Bulloms and Timmanees call this disease kennia, the Mandingos call it corrosilla, and the Soosoos, soogoqúia, or " a sickness caught at night." For the cure, they rely chiefly upon purgative remedies, which are generally of a drastic nature. A number of limes are cut in two, and boiled with water in an iron pot, until one third of the quantity be evaporated : when cool, a cupfull of this decoction is ordered to be taken two or three times a day, or oftener, until it purge briskly. This medicine is violent in its operation, and being continued in the manner they direct, reduces the patient's strength considerably.

Another celebrated remedy for gonorrhœa is obtained from a shrub, called by the Soosoos, bullanta; by the Mandingos, garrágasakkee; by the Bulloms, chuck; and by the Timmanees, tooma. An handful of the leaves is beaten in a mortar with a couple of limes, and the whole is infused for some hours in hot water. Of this infusion the quantity of a tea-cup-full is taken three or four times a day: it is an active purgative without producing much griping. A little of the same infusion is occasionally injected warm into the urethra; it produces but a slight degree of pain. The milky juice of a plant called by the Soosoos, gang-gang; by the Bulloms, semm; and by the Timmanees, prang or owan, proves when taken to the quantity of a large table-spoonfull, violently emetic and purgative without griping, and is frequently used as a cure for gonorrhæa.

In order to abate the ardor urinæ in gonorrhœa, they drink an infusion of the scoparia dulcis; chunkaprum *, (Bullom); karee, (Timmanee): it is taken cold and has a sweet mucilaginous taste.

As an injection they frequently use an infusion of a shrub, called by the Bulloms and Timmanees, nangka; and by the Soosoos, menneh; this is *blown* into the urethra through a small reed, one end of which is inserted into the urethra. Except gonorrhœa I never met with any affection of the urinary passages, such as gravel, calculus, &c. A friend of mine, however, met with an old person, who appeared to be much affected with gravel or stone, and to whom he taught the method of making and using lime water, for which he was very thankful. Mr. Bruce says, " gravel is universally the disease with those who use water from draw wells, as in the desert."

PHLEGMONE TESTIS, swelled testicle, or, as it is

---

* Chunk is the proper name of this shrub, but prum, which signifies a dove in Bullom, is commonly added, because doves feed upon it, and are so remarkably fond of it, that the natives place traps to catch them under these shrubs.

improperly called, hernia humoralis, is not an unfrequent consequence of gonorrhœa, and it appears to be more common among the Foolas, Mandingos, and Soosoos, than among the other nations; owing, perhaps, to the wide and loose drawers which the former people wear. It is observed of the highlanders, that they are very liable to the same complaint, from wearing no breeches; and Mr. Lempriere, in his Tour from Gibraltar to Morocco, speaking of the diseases of the Moors, says, " The cause of hydrocele so frequently occurring in this country, seems to be in a great measure the loose dress of the Moors, and the great relaxation which is induced by the warmth of the climate," to which he adds, " their indulgence in certain pleasures, and the application of the warm bath immediately after." To cure this complaint, the affected part is exposed to the vapour arising from a hot infusion of the leaves of the lime tree, or of those of the bullanta, in water, while the body is covered by a large cotton cloth, to excite a general perspiration. They also use a decoction of a plant called by the Timmanees, améss; and by the Bulloms, nóllee or countopil, which is applied hot, as a fomentation to the part.

A decoction of the three following plants is also administered for the cure of gonorrhœa and swelled testicle, 1. Ronnetookee, (Soosoo). 2. Kundee, called by the Timmanees, kúllepa. 3. Dún-dakka, called by the Timmanees, amelliky.

An infusion of the bark of amelliky is much commended in the cure of gonorrhœa; it is a strong bitter, and acts very powerfully as a diuretic.

The Soosoos frequently employ the root of a vine called kingkréesha, in decoction, as a cure for the venereal disease, but I am uncertain in what stages they use it, or whether it be in gonorrhœa only. It is called by the Bulloms 'n-kay, and by the Timmanees ti-kép. It has a fruit the size of an orange, covered with a thick rind of a yellowish colour, containing a number of large seeds, involved in a white gelatinous matter of an agreeably sweet taste, and frequently eaten by the natives.

An infusion of a plant, called by the Soosoos, nehree; by the Mandingos, nehtee; by the Timmanees, mabie; and by the Bulloms, bee; the mimosa edulis, locust tree; is used in gonorrhœa, and frequently proves emetic. The fruit of this tree is eaten, and soap is made from its ashes.

It has been supposed that in those countries where oil is used in large quantity as an article of diet, herniæ are uncommonly prevalent; this opinion, however, appears to be hypothetical, and founded upon the supposed relaxing properties of oil, rather than upon what really happens, as this disease is by no means so frequent among the Africans as it is among Europeans. I have only seen one instance of it which was of the congenite kind, in a boy about five or six years old. The Soosoos call it kayakái; the Bulloms, kokee.

They do not in general distinguish very accurately between phlegmone testis and hernia: the latter disease is called by the Bulloms, rookra-koonee, rookra signifying the testicle, and koonee the belly: the Soosoos call it quorriakyaky; the Mandingos, contakya; and the Timmanees call it grotoorakoor akoor. They employ the bark of a tree called cup-a-cup which is beaten small, moistened with water, and applied warm as a cataplasm to the tumor. This is repeated several times a day; at the same time an infusion of the same bark is administered internally, though it does not appear with what view this is done, as the bark has no other sensible effects than those of an astringent: brisk purgatives are also occasionally administered. The natives have an idea, that if cold water be poured upon the head in this disease it would be attended with fatal effects.

The COUP DE SOLEIL, or sun stroke, is very common in the hot countries of Europe, and in the southern provinces of America; yet, notwithstanding the long continued and excessive heat of the climate, it is a disease entirely unknown to the Africans. They expose the head uncovered to the perpendicular rays of a scorching sun, during the greatest bodily exertions, with perfect impunity; and children not a month old are exposed, whilst sleeping behind their mothers backs, to the full heat and glare of sunshine, without appearing to suffer in the least. This probably depends upon the great relaxation of the system, by which a general, and profuse perspiration immediately follows the least exertion, and which tends, by promoting an equable circulation, to prevent local congestions in the brain and other viscera, at the same time that it cools the surface by evaporation. The great uniformity in the state of the atmosphere has also a powerful effect : a greater or less degree of haze generally prevails in it, which, without intercepting the rays of heat, renders them more steady and uniform in their effects. The coup de soleil appears to prevail chiefly in those countries where the alternations of heat and cold are considerable, and where the atmosphere is occasionally obscured by clouds ; a portion of this moveable curtain being, for a moment, suddenly removed, the rays of the sun are concentrated as in the focus of a burning lens. It is said that in the year 1743, between the 14th and 25th of July, upwards of eleven thousand persons perished in the streets of Pekin from this cause.

Even Europeans are not liable to sun strokes in Africa, though it be common to see sailors rowing boats during the hottest season, with no other protection from the sun's rays than a thin handkerchief folded round the head, the rest of their dress consisting only of a pair of trowsers. Where Europeans are said to die from this cause in Africa, and perhaps it may be added in the West India Islands, it is usually in consequence of the brain being affected with inflammation from the abuse of those destructive liquors ardent spirits. Persons in an infirm state of health who expose themselves for a considerable time to the rays of the sun, sometimes feel a considerable degree of fulness and tightness in the head, accompanied with a pulsation of the vessels of the brain, so strong that it is heard by the patient: this is followed by no other bad consequences than a severe head-ach, and may be removed by retiring into the shade, using a half erect posture, and occasionally folding a cloth round the head wetted with cold water or vinegar and water.

In the Recueil de Questions proposées à une Societè de Savants, Professor Michaelis asks if pains of the teeth, and decayed teeth, be more rare in Arabia than in Europe; as he entertained an opinion that the use of coffee may have produced a considerable change in the teeth, and may have occasioned disorders in them which were nearly unknown before. The natives of Africa, though they have fine teeth, yet are frequently affected with TOOTH-ACH, and very willingly have recourse to Europeans to have them extracted, an art of which they are totally ignorant. Tooth-ach is called by the Bulloms, kot nekkeeay; and by the Timmanees, attunk arrobang.

The Foolas, owing to their constantly rubbing them, have very decayed teeth, and tooth-ach is just as common among them as it is in England.

The juice of the gang-gang, Soosoo, or milk tree, called by the Timmanees prang, is recommended as a cure for tooth-ach. A few drops of this juice are diluted with water and rubbed upon the gums, and a single drop is put into the tooth when hollow, with the view of destroying the nerve. It is with the juice of this acrid plant that the Foolas poison their arrows: a single drop introduced into the eye excites most excruciating pain, and is followed by loss of sight. The inner part of the bark of the red water tree is sometimes scraped fine, and applied to the gums in tooth-ach; it is very acrid, and when chewed produces some degree of torpor, or slight paralysis of the tongue.

An infusion of a plant, called by the Timmanees talánee, is used warm to wash the mouth; this is frequently repeated; they also inhale the steam of it when boiling. A decoction of the same plant is drank in pains of the bowels.

A decoction of the dried leaves of a plant, called by the Timmanees anúnt, is frequently used warm, to gargle the mouth in pains of the teeth and gums.

APTHOUS ULCERATIONS of the mouth and gums, attended with a spongy and bleeding state of the latter, and looseness of the teeth, are cured by a gargle composed of a decoction of the leaves of kankeebómbo, Soosoo; it is used likewise against pains of the teeth. Scurvy is a disease with which the Africans are wholly unacquainted. Dr. Trotter observes, " From all my enquiries I was not able to learn that such a disease as scurvy was ever seen among the natives of Africa *on shore;* but I verily believe it has occurred more

frequently in Guineamen than has been supposed *."

For PAINS OF THE EAR, the leaves of a plant,
called by the Timmanees kakak, are bruised, and
after being infused in hot water are used as a
fomentation.

DYSENTERY is one of the scourges with which
ships in the slave trade are frequently punished,
causing them to lose a considerable part of their
unfortunate cargo. When the disease prevails
on board these vessels, crowded as they are
with slaves, language is inadequate to convey a
just idea of the loathsome state to which the
poor wretches are reduced. A surgeon of a
Guineaman, describing the mortality which occurred among the slaves, says, " out of the car-
goes of several vessels, consisting of six or seven
hundred (slaves) each, one buried two hundred
and fifty, one two hundred and twenty, one an
hundred and fifty, one sixty, and our ship eighty-
two slaves, most part of them having died of this
terrible disorder †." Philips in his voyage to Guinea informs us, that out of a cargo of seven hundred slaves which he took on board, three hundred and twenty died of different diseases before
he reached Barbadoes, which, he humanely observes, " was to his great regret, after enduring
much misery and stench so long among a parcel
of creatures, nastier than swine : no goldfiner,
he adds, can suffer such noisome drudgery as they

* Observations on the Scurvy.
† Ed. Med. Com. vol. ix. Dec. 1.

do, who carry negroes, having no respite from their afflictions so long as any of their slaves are alive."

A young man, who has no immediate prospect of settling in his profession, is often allured by fair promises to become surgeon of a Guinea ship; but ere long the bright prospect vanishes, and he finds that he has been cruelly deceived, and deplores, when too late, his degrading situation. If he possesses sensibility, his feelings are constantly on the rack; if his constitution be weak, his health is ruined, and he narrowly escapes with life. His attention to the poor creatures under his care must be unremitted; in fact, when sickness prevails he must almost wholly reside between decks, in their place of confinement, where the temperature is about 100° of Fahrenheit's scale, and where " the effluvia are so intolerable, that in a few minutes you may have the condensed vapour from your face in great quantity. He is not always at liberty to exert his medical talents, but must implicitly obey the orders of the captain, who, having made several voyages to the coast, presumes upon his being competent to the cure of all their diseases. Thus, when he has toiled night and day, when his mind is harassed with distress, and his body exhausted with fatigue, if, notwithstanding his utmost efforts, sickness continues to prevail, the master of the vessel, whose character is perfectly congenial to the trade, attributes every misfortune to the machinations of the doctor and devil*."

* Trotter's Observations on Scurvy.

During my residence at Sierra Leone, several instances occurred of surgeons of vessels in the slave trade being obliged to *run away* from their ships, owing to the cruel treatment they had received; and in one instance, which I witnessed, the chief and second mates, surgeon, and several of the crew, were obliged to take refuge in the colony from the fury of their persecutor.

This picture, which is drawn neither through prejudice nor malice, will, it is hoped, render medical men cautious how they engage in this iniquitous traffic; and if attended to, may prevent some aged parent from having his grey hairs brought with sorrow to the grave by the untimely loss of a darling son, or, what is still more to be dreaded, from seeing him return with a depraved heart and a ruined constitution.

Dysentery is by no means so prevalent a disease to the northward of Sierra Leone * as upon the Gold Coast, where the badness of the water renders it very frequent. The natives of the Gold Coast have the credit of being very successful in the cure of this complaint. The chief medicine which they use in it is lime juice, to which is added some of their favourite capsicum or red pepper: this latter is so highly esteemed by them,

* Les habitans de Quoia assurent qu'ils ne savoient autrefois ce que cétoit que la dissenterie; & quelle est venuë chez eux de Sierra Liona. L'an 1626, huit mois après le depart de l' admiral Lam, cette maladie se repandit dans le royaume de Sierra Liona & les pais circonvoisins, & fit de si grands ravages que le terre demeura plus de trois ans sans culture, chacun pensant plus a mourir qu'a se fournier de vivres.' Dapper Descr. de l' Afrique.

that it is used not only as a seasoning to their food, but enters largely into the composition of their medicines, and always constitutes the chief ingredient in their enemas. Marchais[*] says, " on the Gold Coast the cure of colic is a *calabash of lime juice* mixed with red pepper, and drank night and morning for several days:" in pains of the stomach, he adds, " they bind it tight with a cord." Their mode of administering an enema is by means of a gourd scooped hollow, the small end of which is inserted into the anus, and by means of a long small tube fixed to the opposite end of the gourd, the contained fluid is *blown* into the rectum : this operation is generally performed by some old woman, whose services in this way are often called for by Europeans.

In the neighbourhood of Bassa, and upon the Kroo coast, they use for the cure of diarrhœa and dysentery a plant which they call doy, and which the Timmanees call amelliky; nauclea sambucina. A few of the leaves are eaten together with a little Malaguetta pepper, after which some warm water is drank. This remedy is highly extolled by them.

To remove the tormina which occur in dysentery, they use a warm infusion of a plant, called by the Foolas, malanga; by the Soosoos, melleè ; and by the Timmanees and Bulloms, nangka.

But their most celebrated remedy, and one which deserves more particular attention from Europeans, is the bark of a large tree, called by

[*] Voyage en Guinée.

the Foolas, béllenda; and by the Soosoos and Mandingos, bèmbee; rondeletia africana. It is employed either in powder mixed with boiled rice, or is used in a strong infusion. This bark is an agreeable astringent, possessing somewhat of a sweetish taste.

A quantity of this bark was sent to me at Free Town, from the Rio Nunez, where it had been used with very great success in an epidemic dysentery which prevailed among the slaves in the factories of that river. I had not an opportunity of trying its effects in dysentery, as a case of that disease did not occur in the colony from the time I received the bark until I left the country; but in several instances of diarrhœa it shewed itself very effectual. After my arrival in London I gave some of it to my friend Dr. Willan, who made trial of it in agues, fevers, sore throat and dysentery, very much to his satisfaction.

PAINS OF THE BOWELS, somewhat resembling colic, frequently occur among the natives In the month of December 1793, upwards of thirty of the natives were suddenly affected at Bance Island, in the river Sierra Leone, with a species of colic, probably arising from the badness of the water, though they attributed it to the effects of witchcraft. In all these cases bitters are the remedies to which they have recourse.

An infusion of the bark of argol (Timmanee), coontang (Bullom), is much celebrated, taken internally; it is likewise applied hot as a fomentation to the belly.

A decoction of the bark of tookúndoo (Timmanee) is employed in pains of the bowels. This is a powerful bitter, and is taken every morning sweetened with honey; it proves gently purgative : the Bulloms call it lakóona.

The leaves of tokakellee (Soosoo), bruised and infused in cold water, are used in griping pains of the bowels. The infusion is very rough and astringent, and proves gently emetic and purgative.

The water which oozes from the trunk of the plantain when divided, is astringent, and is sometimes employed in diarrhœa.

An infusion of the dried bark of sangbanee (Timmanee), is used in griping pains of the bowels.

A warm infusion of the inner bark (liber) of rómday (Timmanee) dried and powdered, is used in this complaint.

When these pains of the bowels are accompanied with frequent griping stools, a decoction of the fresh root of a plant, called by the Timmanees afoam, is mixed with boiled rice, and taken night and morning.

The root of bèndeky (Soosoo), arrhee (Timmanee) is scraped fine and boiled in water; it is a pretty strong bitter, and much used in pains of the bowels. When the decoction is made strong, the quantity of an ordinary teacupfull proves purgative, without exciting griping.

A decoction of nassum (Timmanee) is also recommended in this complaint and proves gently opening, as also does a decoction of the root of a plant called by the Soosoos whee-yúng-yay, and by the Bulloms lok.

The Soosoos cure pains of the bowels by a decoction of a grass which they call toóngee; the same is also celebrated as a cure for impotency in men.

In colic pains a little of the bark of a tree, called by the Timmanees obéck, and by the Mandingos borrakillee, previously dried in the sun and powdered, is sprinkled upon the rice which they eat at their meals.

The Soosoos frequently use the following curious remedy, they take two leaves of a plant called koomesó-so; by the Timmanees, bia-by; and two leaves of another plant called in Soosoo aboossoo, in Timmanee makunt, which are first bruised and then infused in water, wherein three lighted coals, or rather pieces of ignited charcoal, have been quenched; the water is then poured off and drank.

The Africans do not in general make use of very complex remedies, but the following, which is an exception, is greatly celebrated by the Soosoos, and in the number of ingredients may almost vie with the most celebrated compositions of antiquity* : the leaves of 1. Tengbay. 2. Ballica-

* The mithridate was at first composed of no more ingredients, than the above African remedy; it is said to have con-

sooree-sooree. 3. Morkay or Tamarind. 4. Kan-
keebombay. 5. Quorree. 6. Kebbay. 7. Koo-
lee-yim-ma-bay. 8. Nintee. 9. Morronday.
10. Whee-yung-yay : all boiled in rice water, and
used as common drink for the cure of pains of the
bowels attended with feverish symptoms.

sisted only of twenty leaves of rue, two walnuts, two figs, and
a little common salt.

> Bis denas rutæ frondes, salis & breve granum,
> Juglandesque duas totidem cum corpore ficus.

CHAP. IV.

GENERAL DISEASES.

ELEPHANTIASIS.

ELEPHANTIASIS, or lepra Arabum, has been so called from the resemblance which the diseased skin, particularly that of the legs and feet, bears to the tuberculous, chopped, and rugged hide of an elephant. This similitude has been rather fancifully extended by Aretæus in his elegant and accurate description of this disease. It is moreover called leontiasis, from the thickened state of the eyebrows, and the rugose appearance of the forehead, especially towards the temples and angles of the eyes, which was compared to the countenance of a lion when enraged. Celsus calls it elephantia, and by others it is termed elephas*. The Arabians made a distinction between elephantia or elephantiasis, and elephas; in the former, the disease is spread over the body, in the latter, it is confined to the leg, which becomes enlarged, with varicose veins, a great thickening of the skin, and a prodigious deposition in the adipose membrane. This dreadful disease which at one time excited such a general

---

* Lucretius ; Est elephas morbus, &c.

alarm in modern Europe, frequently occurs in Africa, where, according to the testimony of the ancients, it primarily originated. Lucretius says of it

——————— propter flumina Nili
Gignitur, Ægypto in medio, neque præterea usquam *.

Pliny says the elephantiasis did not appear in Italy before the time of Pompey the Great, and that it was brought thither from Egypt; to which country, the same author adds, the disease is peculiar. As the complaint began in the face, and disfigured the whole visage, but particularly the nose †, it excited general consternation; however, the disease was at that time soon eradicated from Italy. In the Mosaic writings, only that species of the disease is described which is called leuce, consisting of " insensible white spots, smooth, shining, and not elevated ‡." The opinion that it originated in Egypt seems confirmed by its being called the botch of Egypt. It was carried from thence by the Israelites into the land of Canaan, where it probably was not before

* VI. 1112.

† ——————— a facie sæpius incipientem, in nare primum veluti lenticul: mox inarescente per totum corpus, maculosa, variis coloribus, & inæquali cute, alibi crassa, alibi tenui, dura alibi, ceu scabie aspera: ad postremum vero nigrescente, & ad ossa carnes apprimente, intumescentibus digitis in pedibus manibusque. Ægypti peculiare hoc malum: & quum in reges incidisset, populis funebre. Quippe in balineis solia temperabantur humano sanguine ad medicinam eam.

‡ Dr. Willan's Lectures. Plin. lib. 26. c. v.

known. From Palestine it was brought into Europe by those who returned from the crusades. Upon its first introduction into Europe this disease spread with astonishing rapidity; in the ninth century there were throughout Christendom 19000 hospitals for lepers. In the year 1227, Lewis VIII. king of France, bequeathed legacies to 2000 hospitals for leprous patients in his own kingdom, which was one third less than it is at present. This is not a solitary instance of a new disease making suddenly an almost universal ravage, and in process of time becoming milder. A similar progress was observed in the venereal disease. The small pox likewise, when first carried to America, was infinitely more destructive than in Europe, from whence it was imported, than it is in America at the present day. It may be further remarked, that in the time of Moses the disease must have been quicker in its progress than it is at the present time, since the changes which occurred in seven, or at most in fourteen days, were thought sufficient to decide upon the nature of the disease.

This disease appeared in the island of Java about the year 1661, where it seems to have been introduced and diffused by contagion. A predisposition to it was supposed to have been formed by the diet of the inhabitants, consisting of salt, putrid fish, and other indigestible foods, with high seasonings of every kind, but especially pepper; this they eat by handfuls, " atque ad libidinis pruritum excitandum aro quotidie in cibis utuntur *.'

The first well marked case of the disease, which occurred to me in Africa, was that of a Foola man named Mamadoo Minnioo Casoo, who came with Mr. Watt and my brother from Calleesar, near Teembo, to seek medical advice at Sierra Leone. This person was about 50 years of age, tall and thin, but muscular, and had a very great flow of spirits. The only visible appearance of disease in him consisted in several discolourations of the skin, of an irregular figure, rather larger than a crown piece, and of a light copper colour †. These discoloured patches were upon

---

* Bonetus Medic. Septent. lib. vi.

† This disease is very frequent in the French colony of Cayenne, where, from the coppery appearance of the diseased skin, it bears the name of *mal rouge*. It affects the European as well as negro inhabitants, but more frequently the latter, and is held in the utmost horror by all. The chief diagnostics of this diease are thus described by Bajon Nachrichten zur Geschichte von Cayenne. The spots are not circumscribed, or well defined ; they are not of a bright red ; they are extensively spread over the body, and mixed with yellow spots ; they appear upon the forehead, ears, hands, shoulders, loins, legs, and feet, and although they may have been of long standing, they still continue to spread. But the symptom most to be depended on is their insensibility. If on the contrary a person be affected with spots or patches, which are of a lively red, and bounded by a circle of a still higher colour ; if while they spread, the middle of the spots reassumes the natural colour of the skin ; if they be sensible, and especially if attended with violent itching, they are not symptoms of the mal rouge, but merely of herpes. Besides the mal rouge, Professor Sprengel enumerates the following as varieties of lepra : 1. The northern leprosy, in Norway termed radeseuche ; in Iceland, liktraa. 2. The disease of the Crimea. 3. The Aleppo boil. 4. The erisipelas of Asturia. 5. Pellagra.

the arms, trunk of the body and legs. Owing to the different shades of their colour contrasted with the black skin, the spots appeared slightly elevated round the edges, though this was not perceptible to the touch. When the finger was slightly rubbed over them, they felt rather smoother than the other parts of the skin, which, however, was as soft and smooth as the skins of the Africans are in general. When closely viewed with a small convex lens, these discolourations did not appear to differ from the texture of the surrounding sound skin, nor did there appear to be the slightest elevation in them. The number of patches upon the trunk were six, the same number upon the arms, and as many upon the legs and thighs.

A very slight change of colour had taken place upon the edge of the upper lip, near the angle of the mouth, but so trifling that it would perhaps have escaped my notice had he not pointed it out himself. A very small part of the right ala nasi likewise appeared thickened and discoloured.

The parts of the skin, thus discoloured, were totally devoid of sensibility, which the man noticed himself, saying he could not feel if they were either cut or pinched. When a pin was run through these discoloured spots he complained of no pain until it touched the muscular parts below.

The disease was of eight years standing when I saw him; it made its first appearance on the outside of the fore arm, but he did not notice it until after he had received a smart blow upon the part, though he did not attribute the disease to this cause. After the patch upon the arm had acquired nearly its present size, almost two years elapsed without his observing any further appearance of disease. At the end of this time a similar appearance took place upon the outside of the leg, which continued to increase very gradually in size; and a twelvemonth elapsed without his perceiving any further increase of 'the disease. Two large patches then shewed themselves upon the right breast, one above, the other below the nipple; about the same time other discolourations appeared upon the trunk, legs, and arms, at first small, but gradually increasing in size. No new spots have appeared for two or three years past until about three months ago, when the ala nasi became affected, and about two months since it made its appearance upon the lip. These last appear to him to increase in size, but the others seem nearly stationary.

He feels no pain nor uneasiness, except at times slight formications over his body in different parts of the skin. His appetite is very good and all the functions natural. He has had four children, who all died before he became affected with this disease. His wife, with whom he still cohabits, is not affected, nor has she, he says, any apprehension of catching the disorder. By ancient writers this complaint has been called saty-

riasis, ob inexplebilem coeundi libidinem*. This
was denied by my patient, who said it did not
occur in his country to those affected like him;
but he appeared a little offended that a diminu-
tion of his powers should be suspected.

This person was remarkably communicative,
and possessed a cultivated mind. He informed
me that this disease is very frequent in the Foola
country, where it is greatly dreaded on account
of the horrid ravages it makes upon the bodies
of those affected with it. They consider it as a
disorder admitting of long life, but that it ulti-
mately proves fatal. They use several remedies,
chiefly infusions of vegetables taken internally and
applied as baths, but seem to receive little advantage from any of them. They consider this disorder
as hereditary, though the offspring of deceased parents are not always affected with it, but sometimes
escape during their life; and they are rarely or never affected with the disease until after puberty.
He mentioned an instance of a man whom he knew,
whose hands had dropped off at the wrists in consequence of this disease, and who had married a
woman afflicted with the same complaint, though
in a less degree, no other being willing to marry
him. They had from this marriage three sons,
who are now alive and grown up, but only one of
them is affected with elephantiasis.

* By Galen it is also called satyriasmos, from the face being
made to resemble that of a satyr.

Although the disease be not always regular in its appearance and progress, they distinguish three species of it, to each of which they give a distinct name. The first is called by the Foolas, dama-dyang; by the Soosoos, dhay; and by the Man-dingos, koonah: this is commonly the first appearance of the disease, and is the mildest form in which it appears. The skin is merely discoloured and insensible, as in the case above-mentioned.

2. Didyam*, called by the Soosoos quolla karree, and by the Mandingos baghèè. In this species the disease is more advanced; in addition to the insensibility and discolouration of the skin, the joints of the fingers and toes are affected with spreading ulcerations; they become considerably enlarged, and at length drop off. The lobes of the ears are much thickened and enlarged, and discharge a thick viscid matter. The lips are much swoln, and the alæ nasi are tumefied and ulcerated. The first species of this disease is sometimes cured, or rather checked in its progress, by art or nature. The second also, though more rarely, is sometimes prevented from spreading.

The third species is called barras; by the Soosoos, daghee; and by the Mandingos, daa. This stage of the disorder is chiefly characterized by the voice, which becomes hoarse and guttural, the patient usually speaking through his nose, as in ozæna, because of the great and spreading ulcer-

---

* This word is sometimes written sghidam; and by Niebuhr, dsjuddam or madsjurdam.

ation in the throat and fauces. The progress of
the disease is now very rapid, and when the voice
becomes nearly unintelligible, death is supposed
to be not far distant*. Together with the affection of the throat and nose, the neck is much
tumefied; the ears are more and more ulcerated,
the legs and feet, deprived of the toes, enlarge
greatly, and entirely lose their form. The whole
of the skin is also much thickened, and affected in
various parts with foul ulcerations. The species of
the disease, called alopecia, is unknown here : the
beard and hair upon other parts of the body
are neither changed in their colour nor fall off,
though the parts upon which they grow be discoloured by the disease. In the patient above-
mentioned, his face not being affected where the
beard grows, and those parts of his body where
the discolourations were, being quite smooth, it
afforded no opportunity to observe what change
the hair would have undergone.

There is a disease called by the Soosoos yábba
séray, which appears from the description of the
natives to be a variety of barras. It is said not
to be infectious; it appears first in numerous
small pustules about the neck or arms, spreading
from thence to various parts of the body. When
scratched, the pimples came off in scales, and

---

* This stage of the disease is very accurately described by
Galen : ' Elephas, est affectus qui cutem crassam atque inequabilem
reddit, livor adest tum cuti, tum oculorum albis, exeduntur
partes manuum, ac pedum summæ, ex quibus sanies livida, ac
fœtida emanat. Galeni Isag. 172.

they sometimes discharge a little watery fluid. If the skin of the affected part be cut, no blood issues, nor is any pain felt. These eruptions produce intolerable itching, which is not increased by being in bed or in the cold. When they affect the head, the hair is changed to a dirty white, and falls off. The disease is said to be curable if taken in time, but its appearance always excites a great alarm. It does not affect either hands or feet, and is said to prove fatal in little more than a year. It sometimes produces a tumefaction of the nose, lips, and ears, but never affects the throat.

As my patient staid only a few days at Free Town, being obliged to return with the embassador sent by the Foola king, I had not an opportunity of trying the effects of medicine; nor could I venture to trust him with an active remedy, where a mistake in the dose, &c. might have been attended with unpleasant consequences, I gave him therefore a bottle of vin. antimon. with directions to take a tea-spoonful twice a day; and some flor. sulphur. to take occasionally as a laxative, hoping that, as it affects the odour of the perspiration it might also act upon the skin *. Had he continued for any length of time,

* Niebuhr says that a negro, who had been attacked at Mokha with the species of leprosy called bohak, which, he adds, is neither contagious nor fatal; and perhaps resembled that of the Foola above-mentioned, except in the colour of the spots, which were white. His complaint was alleviated for a time, though not cured, by the use of sulphur.

it was my wish to have tried the mineral solution
(of arsenic*) and in case of failure of success to
have used the julep. sublimat. notwithstanding the
use of mercury is condemned in this disease †.

Upon the island of Bananas I saw two other
cases of elephantiasis ; in one, a man, the leg was
chiefly affected, being much tumefied, the skin
thick, hard, and deeply furrowed, though without
any ulceration or discharge ; the toes were not
affected. In the other case, a woman of middle
age, who had laboured under the disease several

* Arsenic is considered as a specific in this disease by the Hin-
doo physicians, among whom it has long been a secret remedy.
Its preparation is thus described : " Take of white arsenic, fine and
fresh, one tolà (or the weight of 105 grains troy) ; of picked black
pepper six times as much ; let both be well beaten at intervals,
for four days successively, in an iron mortar, and then reduced to
an impalpable powder in one of stone with a stone pestle, and
thus completely levigated, a little water being mixed with them,
make pills of them as large as tares or small pulse, and keep them
dry in a shady place. One of these pills must be swallowed
morning and evening with some *betel* leaf, or in countries where
betel is not at hand, with cold water : if the body be cleansed
from foulness and obstructions by gentle cathartics and bleeding
before the medicine is administered, the remedy will be speedier."
An instance is given of a cure being obtained in three weeks by
the above plan. Asiat. Researches, vol. ii.

† About two years afterwards this old man paid a second visit
to Free Town ; he was much pleased with his medicines, which
he had taken with great regularity, and even flattered ·himself
that he had got rid of his complaint ; but after eating some kind
of food which had disagreed with him, he had been affected with
a swelling of his belly, from which he recovered with some difficulty. After this, his former complaint returned, and when I saw
him his fingers had become affected with slight ulcerations, especially about the roots and edges of his nails. The discoloured
patches had suffered no material change, nor had any fresh ones
appeared.

years, the face was the part chiefly affected,
though the skin of her whole body was rugose and
much thickened. Her voice was very hoarse, and
her throat, on inspection, appeared inflamed with
erysipelatous inflammation, but not ulcerated.
With respect to the general appearance and deformity of her countenance, she much resembled a
person in the most confluent small pox when
the face is most swoln, though the tubercles on
her face were not numerous, nor much elevated
above the skin. This was the only instance which
occurred to me that bore any resemblance to the
facies leonina of authors. Her hair was not in
the least altered, neither were the joints of her
fingers or toes affected. There were no discoloured patches visible upon her skin. She was
wife to a very celebrated man, well known by the
title of Lord North, and conscious of her dignity,
she did not like to be too closely examined.

Another instance of this disease, in a woman
about forty years of age, came under my notice.
The chief appearance consisted in irregular patches
of a light copper colour spread over her body,
especially upon the breast; these parts were perfectly insensible when the skin was pierced by a
pin. She had lost some of the joints of her fingers
and toes, but they were healed when I saw her,
and did not shew any disposition to break out
again. She had borne two children since the
spots first appeared.

A slave trader, who had been brought up to
medicine, informed me that he had seen three

instances of elephantiasis in the Mandingo country, two of which were men* and one a woman.
In all these cases, the disease shewed itself by
discolourations of the skin, which were followed
by tumefaction, and ulceration of the fingers and
toes, all of which at length dropped off. In the
woman, the disease appeared to be subdued,
or to have received a check during the space of
two years that she resided at his factory; this he
attributed to her having a more nourishing diet,
while with him, than she had been accustomed
to before. Another case of this disease occurred
to myself at a town belonging to Manga Dooba,
near the False Cape (Sierra Leone). The patient
was a young man, about twenty-two years of age,
tall, and of a robust form; he had been affected
with elephantiasis for several years. Neither his
father nor mother, nor any of his relations as far
as he could remember, had been ever afflicted
with this disease. One striking peculiarity occurred in this person; almost the whole of his
skin had suffered a change of colour from black
to a very light brown or copper colour. Very
little of the original colour now remained, except
one large spot round the umbilicus, and another
upon his back and legs. Every part of his body
was sensible when pricked with a pin. He had

---

* It is said by Piso, that men are more subject to elephantiasis
than women, which accords very well with my experience; De
Cognosc. & Cur. Morb. iii. 63. The same has also been remarked
by Archigenes: Apprehenduntur autem hac affectione viri magis
quam feminæ. Ætii Tetrab. 4. s. i. c. 120.

lost the first joints of the thumb, fore, and little
fingers of his right hand; and also the first and
second joints of the thumb, and of all the fingers
of the left hand. The remaining joint of the ring
finger of the left hand was much swoln, though
he said it was subsiding, that finger having been
the one last affected. The ends of the stumps
of the fingers were all healed over, but had all of
them small conical projections like the end of a
sugar loaf. The fingers and toes are always
much swoln, and almost lose their form before
they ulcerate and drop off, or before the disease
cuts them, as they term it; but this tumefaction
very soon afterwards subsides. He complained
of much pain in his fingers and feet, especially
towards night; his toes were not affected, but his
ancles were rather enlarged, and bore the marks
of large ulcers upon them, which were now healed
up. The edges of these cicatrices appeared of a
darker colour than the middle part, and seemed
to be somewhat raised and puckered all round.
His skin appeared in many parts very foul, as if
from cutaneous eruptions just healed, but was not
covered with scales. These defœdations were
chiefly visible upon the arms, legs, and neck;
other parts of his skin, though changed from their
original colour, still retained their smoothness.
Several little pustules containing a whitish fluid,
were observable about his shoulders, which he said
broke out into superficial ulcerations and healed
after some time, leaving an ugly scar behind.
Upon the fore finger of the right hand was one

of these ulcerations, which at first view appeared
as if the cuticle had been accidentally abraded,
but upon a closer inspection the edges appeared
covered with a foul thin crust. This man was
not, at the time, under any course of medicine,
nor did he make any application to the sores:
cow's dung is most commonly used as a plaister
for them. A year had elapsed since his fingers
dropped off, and the disease did not appear
when I saw him to be making any further
progress. Neither his face nor throat were affected, nor was his hair in the least altered.
He was remarkably cheerful and active, dancing,
tumbling, and running about with the most perfect unconcern.

When the disease has been stationary for a
length of time, these discolourations frequently
begin to disappear, and the skin gradually regains
its former sensibility. They look upon the disease as cured or put a stop to, as soon as the
skin has recovered its pristine hue, and expect a
return of the disease only when the skin again
changes its colour. At Wankapong, in the Soosoo country, I saw a man who had lost the fingers
and thumbs of both his hands by the elephantiasis,
and all his toes except the great ones *. Discoloured
patches had appeared in various parts of his body
at the commencement of the disease, and conti-

* —— sæpe hominem paullatim cernimus ire,
Et membratim vitalem deperdere sensum :
In pedibus primum digitos livescere, & ungueis,
Inde pedes, & crura mori: post inde per artus
Ire alios tractim gelidi vestigia lethi. Lucr. lib. 3. 525.

nued during the whole of its progress, but when I saw him, 1796, they had disappeared, his skin being of the natural colour, and smooth. The disease had begun ten years before I saw him, but during the last six years it had become stationary, and he considered himself cured, without apprehending any relapse. Some people complain, that in these discoloured places, though insensible to the prick of a pin, there is occasionally great pain, which they compare to the sensation excited by boiling water, or the application of a red hot iron.

This disease does not appear to be so common among the Bulloms and Timmanees as among the Mandingos and Foolas, &c. neither do the former distinguish the different stages of the complaint. The Bulloms call it ghell, and the Timmanees, arroom. When affected with this disease they abstain from eating the flesh of the wild hog, but eat freely of every other kind of food. They appear to follow the advice of Aretæus, in using many and various remedies; but with him also they consider the disease as incurable *. They, however, assert, that a people who live ' far, very far inland,' in a country called Bamballee, pro-

---

* In the West Indies, " the leprosy, the most dreadful of all diseases, is said to have its indigenous remedy, known to few besides the Aborigines of the islands. This remedy, I am informed, is the saururus cernuus of Linnæus, the herb à colet, and aguarima of M. Desportes. The Caribs are said to use it successfully, externally and internally, in this deplorable disease." Chisholm on the Fever of Grenada.

bably Bambarra, can cure it ; but this rests upon no firmer foundation than their idea respecting man-eaters, a denomination applied by them to people living at the same distance, and of whom they have as little knowledge.

Although the flesh of snakes be frequently eaten by the natives of Africa, it is not taken in a medical view, nor have they an idea of any medicinal powers in these reptiles. The ancients were firmly persuaded that such food possessed uncommon virtues, and Pliny attributes the longevity of the inhabitants of Mount Athos, who he says reached the advanced age of 140 years, to their eating vipers. The Greek physicians also attributed to this diet very wonderful effects, and recommended it as a certain cure for elephantiasis; Galen * in particular, has recorded several instances of its efficacy, and gives particular directions for its preparation. In South America lizards are strongly recommended in the cure of cancer, and several instances are recorded of their wonderful effects in this and other diseases. " They cut off the head and tail of the animal, take out its entrails, skin it, chew it, and swallow it directly, while still bloody, warm, and in some degree alive." It is about eight or ten inches long, and probably is the same with the small brown lizards, which inhabit dwelling houses within the tropics. From one to three each day is a proper dose. The patient feels a considerable

* Galen de Arte Cur. lib. ii.

degree of heat over the whole body after eating
the lizard, followed by sweating and a degree of
salivation. It might be worth while to make
trial of this simple remedy in the elephantiasis, as
we have hitherto none which can be depended on
in this dreadful disease *. Vide Aetii Tetrabi.
s. ii. c. 170.

The Africans know of no cause to which they
can attribute this disease; and it may be observed, that of all the causes assigned by authors,
there is none which can be deemed perfectly satisfactory. Climate, diet, and suppression of perspiration from cold, have been considered as the principal causes. But we find that this disease occurs in
a great variety of climates†, even in the finest
of the world. It takes place in nations using
the most opposite modes of diet; it is found
more frequently in warm than in cold climates; nor do we find in England that glass-
makers, who are perhaps more than others exposed to the effects of suppressed perspiration,
are peculiarly liable to this disease. Eunuchs are
said not to be affected with it, which has occasioned some to have recourse to the operation of castration ‡. Piso says, " castratio præterea, ut *singulare remedium,* antiquis probata
est §."

* Ed. Med. Com. Dec. II. vol. v.
† Regio vero hujus mali inductrix est tum quæ valde calida
est, tum quæ vehementer frigida est. Aetii Tetrabibli iv. sermo i.
c. 120.
‡ Mangeti Bibl. Chir. ii. 16.
§ Piso de cognosc. & cur. Morbis, lib. iii. c. 63.

Neque enim temere reperias, inquit Archigenes, ullum aliquem castratum elephantiasi laborantem, neque item facile mulierem. Aetii Tetrab. iv. ser. i. c. 120. Dr. Rush is of opinion that " the leprosy, elephantiasis, scurvy, and venereal disease, appear to be different modifications of the same primary disorder *. The same causes produce them in every age and country.——They all sprung originally from a moist atmosphere and unwholesome diet : hence we read of their prevailing so much in the middle centuries, when the principal parts of Europe were overflowed with water, and the inhabitants lived entirely on fish, and a few unwholesome vegetables.——The elephantiasis is almost unknown in Europe. The leprosy is confined chiefly to *the low countries of Africa.*" In a note he adds, " the same diet, and the same dampness of soil and air, produced the same effects in South America." These observations do not exactly apply to this disease in Africa : the Foola country, where the elephantiasis is rather more prevalent than upon the low swampy coast, is in general hilly, particularly about Teembo. The land, as has been already said, is well cultivated and clear of wood. The air is remarkably dry, insomuch that the paper, which was so damp in the Rio Nunez as scarce to bear ink, became quite dry and stiff before Mr. Watt and my brother reached Teembo. They could

---

* Elephas, lues venerea, & struma, aliquid habent cognatum & συγγενες, tres has hydras unus alexicacos Hercules hydrargyrosis vincit & opprimit. Ballonii, lib. i. Epid. & Ephem. p. 15.

not prevent the tobacco leaves, which they carried with them, from falling to powder, though it was wetted frequently. Salt continues dry in the open air, and iron, which rusts in a very short time at Sierra Leone, whatever care be taken to prevent it, is not in the least affected when exposed to the air in the Foola country. The water which they drink is excellent.

In the early stages of this disease, the only pathognomonic symptom of it appears to be insensibility of the diseased skin, whether there be tubercles, or merely discoloured patches; but this appears to be carried too far when it is asserted that a sharp instrument may be run to the bone without exciting pain; for as the disease often spreads very slowly, the insensibility is at first probably confined to the skin, and goes deeper by degrees. Other symptoms generally enumerated, as the falling off and change of colour of the hair, the unctuous appearance of the skin, the soreness of the throat, and hoarseness, are not always present, even in the advanced stages of the disease.

A just distinction has not yet been made between lepra and elephantiasis, as the description of these diseases by different authors may be mutually mistaken for each other. It is likewise usual to apply the term lepra to every obstinate eruption of the skin; hence herpes, impetigo, ichthyosis, and a variety of other skin complaints, have been included under it. The same has been done with regard to elephantiasis. Dr. Haller, speaking

of this disease, in which he says " tubercles appear
over all the body, and break out into ill conditioned ulcers corrupting the bones," adds, " is
not this the yaws of the English?" Through inat-
tention, enlargements of the legs, with thickening
of the integuments, from whatever cause they
originated, have been considered as elephantiasis.
Boerhaave enumerates among the symptoms of
the advanced stage of scurvy, sicca & lenis
elephantiasis; and Van Swieten is of opinion that
the elephantiasis as described by Aretæus bears a
great resemblance to scurvy. Dr. Hillary has
committed a similar error in his account of the
diseases of Barbadoes: under the title elephantiasis, he describes very accurately a disease
which is endemial in that island, and therefore
called the Barbadoes leg, but which bears no
other resemblance to the true elephantiasis than
the increase of bulk in the limb. In the West
Indies, elephantiasis is very frequent among the
slaves, by whom it is called cacabay. This is very
well described by Dr. Hillary, under the titles
lepra Arabum, and leprosy of the joints, where,
it is evident, he describes only different stages of
the same disease.

In those countries where this disease occurs
frequently, the natives are much alarmed at the
appearance of any eruption. Mr. Bruce informs
us, that the sight of a pimple upon his body will
give an Abyssinian a serious alarm, and cause
him to keep closely within doors until it disappears.

Notwithstanding the custom which has prevailed among many nations, where elephantiasis is frequent, of secluding from society the unhappy persons affected with this disease, it remains doubtful whether it be ever communicated by contagion *. The Africans deny that it is contagious, and make no scruple to eat out of the same dish, and even to sleep in the same bed with a person labouring under elephantiasis. They likewise assert that it is incapable of being communicated by coition; neither do they believe that it is hereditary, but, they consider it is a sickness sent by God. In the case of the woman whom I saw on the island of Bananas, I was requested not to permit her to breathe upon me : this was, however, evidently occasioned by her disgusting appearance, as those who constantly attended upon her did not harbour any fears of being infected.

From the description of this disease in the Mosaic writings we may collect, that, although it was considered by the Jews as hereditary, they did not think it contagious. For though strictly forbidden by the law, lepers were permitted to

---

* Archigenes observes, " Est autem gravis morbus, & prope ex eorum numero qui incurabiles existunt, & gravis quidem est ipsi ægro, intolerabilis autem conspicientibus, utpote qui ipsum omnino aversantur, adeo ut et plerique ex necessariis & domesticis ægri ipsius conversationem devitent. Etenim suspicionem de se præbet malum tanquam sit contagiosum. Atque ego sanè malum esse affirmo cum ipsis conversari; inquinatur enim aer quem inspirando adtrahimus ex ulcerum fœtore, & ex vitiata spiritus exhalatione. Aetii Tetrab. iv. ser. i. c. 120.

dwell among them; and we find the people
commanded at different times to put out of the
camp " every leper, and every one that hath an
issue, and whosoever is defiled by the dead."
Hence it would appear that they were more
afraid of legal pollution than of infection, otherwise the dread of so loathsome a disease would
have rendered this command unnecessary. Moreover, when this disease is mentioned in the Scrip-
tures, it is generally classed with other things
which they held to be unclean, and would defile
any who touched them. Even the dead bodies of
those who had been affected with it were buried
apart : king Uzziah, after having lived in a separate house, was not even buried in the sepul-
chre of the kings, " because he was a leper."
The curse of David upon Joab was a wish that
there might not be wanting in his house " one
that hath an issue, or that is a leper, or that
leaneth on a staff, or that falleth on the sword, or
that lacketh bread," all which were odious in the
sight of the Jews. The four lepers who sat at the
gate of Samaria during the siege, appear to have
had it in their power to enter either into the city
or the camp of the Syrians; and our Saviour ate in
the house of Simon the leper with his disciples.
Naaman the Syrian we find conversing freely with
his master, which would not have been the case
had there been any dread of infection. Josephus
also observes, that in many nations, lepers were
so far from being despised and shunned, that they
frequently were invested with the highest offices

in the state, and permitted to enter the temples. The Jews knew of no cure for this disease, though some have said that the leprosy of Naaman was cured by the sulphureous quality of the waters of Jordan, and that many received benefit from them in leprous diseases. This, however, is contradicted by our Saviour, who says, " many lepers were in Israel in the time of Elisha the prophet, yet none of them was cleansed but Naaman the Syrian."

Herodotus says, if any of the Persians be affected with lepra, or leuce they can hold no communication with those who are well *.

This disease was considered as contagious by the Greek physicians. Aretæus says, that the miserable patients were banished into deserts, or to the tops of mountains, where the kindness of friends occasionally alleviated their distresses ; though perhaps more frequently they were deserted.   Galen was so fully persuaded of its contagious nature, that he says, a leper having infected some of his friends, the rest, in order to avoid danger, built for him, upon a hill just without the village, a hovel to dwell in, seen by Galen, when a young man, in Asia †.   Cælius Aurelianus, whose description of the symptoms of elephantiasis is lost, a circumstance the more to be regretted, as he was an African, and no doubt had often seen the disease in his own country, ob-

* Clio, 138.   † Lib. ii. de Medic. Simpl. Facult.

serves, " Some advise, that a person labouring under this disease should be turned out of the town if a stranger, or if an inhabitant, be banished to some distant part; others advise the patient to be totally abandoned *."

The Chinese, we are informed by Sir G. Staunton in his Account of the Embassy to China, suppose this disease to be infectious. " It is likely," says this ingenious author, " that the general use of linen, to which Europe is supposed to be indebted for its present exemption from leprous affections, will be adopted by the Chinese, in the course of their increased commerce and connections with Europeans. Leprous disorders are those alone for which any hospitals are regularly erected in China, on the principle of their being too infectious to admit of persons affected with them having any communication with the rest of society."

Mr. Maundrell, in his Journey from Aleppo to Jerusalem, thus describes the leprosy: " When I was in the Holy Land, I saw several that laboured under Gehazi's distemper — particularly at Sichem (now Naplosu) there were no less than ten that came a begging to us at one time. Their manner is to come with small buckets in their hands, to receive the alms of the charitable; their touch being still held infectious, *or at least unclean*. The distemper, as I saw it in them, was very different from what I have seen it in Eng-

* Lib. iv. c. 1.

land ; for it not only defiles the whole surface of
the body with a foul scurf, but also deforms the
joints of the body, particularly those of the wrists
and ankles; making them swell with a gouty
scrophulous substance, very loathsome to look
upon. I thought their legs resembled those of old
battered horses, such as are often seen in drays in
England. The whole distemper indeed, as it there
appeared, was so noisome, that it might well pass
for the utmost corruption of the human body on
this side the grave." Van Egmont says there is
at Damascus an hospital for Turkish lepers, but
adds, " the leprosy here is very different from
that known in our country, the patients being
frightful spectacles ; their sallow ghastly faces,
and small hollow eyes, terrifying the spectator.
This distemper, it seems, penetrates to the very
bone, infecting every part of the body ; and the
only alleviation is frequent bathing *."

Niebuhr describes three species, or rather stages,
of leprosy, which he does not say is infectious.
In some places he informs us they take precautions against this disease; as at Abuschahr, they
send to the island Bahrajn, all those affected
with leprosy, and those who had dangerous venereal complaints. At Basra also, and at Bagdad, lepers were shut up in places appointed;
but this was not observed with much care, as
they were allowed every Friday to ask alms in

* Travels through Europe and Asia Minor, ii. 251.

the public markets *. Mr. Forskal likewise says this disease is not contagious, even if any one sleeps with an infected person. At Damascus, as he was informed, there are two parts of the city appropriated to lepers, one for Mahometans, the other for Christians, in which likewise obstinate venereal complaints are included. As the prisoners marry, when a child is born among them, it is taken from the mother, and given to an healthy nurse. If after three months the child shews no symptoms of leprosy, it is brought up in the city; if the disease appears, it is restored to the parents, and the nurse has no apprehension of being infected from it.

In South America, where this disease is frequent, Don Ulloa informs us it is universally believed to be infectious. " The inhabitants of Carthagena, together with those in the whole extent of its government, are very subject to the mal de san lazaro, or leprosy, which seems still to gain ground. Some physicians attribute the prevalence of it to pork, which is here a very common food; but it may be objected, that in other countries, where this flesh is as frequently eaten, no such effects are seen, whence it evidently appears that some latent quality of the climate must also contribute to it. In order to stop the contagion of this distemper, there is, without the city, an hospital called San Lazaro, not far from the hill, on which is a castle of the

* Niebuhr Descript. de l'Arabie.

same name. In this hospital all persons of both sexes labouring under this distemper are confined, without any distinction to age or rank, and if any refuse to go, they are forcibly carried thither. But here the distemper increases among themselves, they being permitted to intermarry, by which means it is rendered perpetual. Besides, their allowance being here too scanty to subsist on, they are permitted to beg in the city; and from their intercourse with those in health, the number of lepers never decreases, and is at present so considerable, that their hospital resembles a little town. Every person at his entering this structure, where he is to continue during life, builds a cottage, called in this country Bugis, proportional to his ability, where he lives in the same manner as before in his house, the prohibition of not going beyond the limits prescribed to him, unless to ask alms in the city, only excepted. The ground on which the hospital stands is surrounded by a wall, and has only one gate, and that always carefully guarded. Amidst all the inconveniences attending this distemper, they live a long time under it, and some even attain to an advanced age. It also greatly increases the natural desire of coition and intercourse of the sexes; so that, to avoid the disorders which would result from indulging this passion, now almost impossible to be controuled, they are permitted to marry *."

* Ulloa's Voyage to South America.

Dr. Bancroft says, leprosy is very common in Guiana, and is deemed infectious. Those affected with this disease are separated from society. The same author adds, however, that he has known leprous slaves, who have privately cohabited a long time with their former wives during the course of this disease, without communicating the infection. Lepers, he adds, are notorious for their salacity and longevity *.

Dr. Heberden, who had frequent opportunities of observing this disease in the island of Madeira, is of opinion that it is not so contagious as is commonly imagined. He never heard of any one contracting the disease from a leper by contact, though he has witnessed the daily communication of lepers with persons unaffected with the disease. He has also known several instances of leprous husbands cohabiting for several years with healthy women, and having several children by them, without communicating the disease, although the children have inherited it. In such families, some of the children have the disease, while others escape. Dr. Heberden adds, that he knew a family " whose father lived and died a leper; and of two sons and two daughters who survived him, though at present each of them is advanced in years, the youngest daughter alone has shewed she inherits the disorder ; and what I think worthy of remark is, that, although the eldest son, at present between sixty and seventy

* Hist. of Guiana.

years of age, has never discovered in himself the least symptom of it, yet his only daughter, now about eighteen years old, has been affected therewith several years. Thus suppressed, but not subdued, we see that the fomes morbi may lie dormant a whole generation, and awake with full vigour in the succeeding one." Med. Trans. vol. i. p. 32. There appears a striking resemblance between these opinions and those commonly entertained in England respecting scrophula and some other supposed hereditary diseases.

Mr. Savary gives an affecting description of the sufferings of those who labour under this disease, which frequently occurs in the fine climate of Greece, and of the islands of the Archipelago. He says, " it is infectious, and is *instantly* communicated by contact. The victims, who are attacked by it, are driven from society, and confined to little ruinous houses on the highway. They are strictly forbidden to leave these miserable dwellings, or hold intercourse with any person. Those poor wretches have, generally, beside their huts, a small garden, producing pulse, and feeding poultry, and with that support, and what they obtain from passengers, they find means to drag out a painful life, in circumstances of shocking bodily distress. Their bloated skin is covered with a scaly crust, speckled with red and white spots, which afflict them with intolerable itchings. A hoarse and tremulous voice issues from the bottom of their breasts.

Their words are scarce articulated, because their distemper inwardly preys upon the organs of speech. These frightful spectres gradually lose the use of their limbs. They continue to breathe till such time as the whole mass of their blood is corrupted, and their bodies are entirely in a state of putrefaction. No sight can be more painful or shocking than that of a leprous person; no torments are equal to what he endures. The rich are not attacked by this distemper: it con fines itself to the poor *, chiefly to the Greeks,

---

* Prosper Alpinus attributes the frequency of this disease in Egypt to the wretched diet, and stagnant water made use of by the poorer sort of inhabitants. De Medic. Egyptiorum, lib. i. 56.

Galen entertained nearly the same opinion; he says, In Alex· andria quidem elephantis morbo plurimi corripiuntur propter victus modum, & regionis fervorem. At in Germania & Mysia rarissima hæc passio videtur. Et apud Scythas *lactis potatores* nunquam fere apparuit. In Alexandria vero plurimum gene· ratur ex victus ratione. Comedunt enim farinam elixatam, & lentem, & cochleas, & plura salita, & nonnulli ex ipsis carnes asininas, & alia quædam quæ crassum & atræ bilis humorem generant. Nam cum circumstans aer calidus sit, motus humo· rum agitur versus cutem. Huic igitur morbo, quas antea dix· imus conferunt purgationes. Quod si & ætas & victus permiserint, sanguis prius mittendus est. Galeni de Arte Cur. lib. ii.

In Hindostan, where elephantiasis has long been known, and where it rages with great violence, it is attributed to the unwhole- some diet of the natives, who are accustomed, after eating plen- tifully of fish, to swallow large draughts of milk. The use of provocatives is also blamed. This disease is said to be extremely contagious, and to be hereditary. It is thought to be the judham (or juzam, as the word is pronounced in India) of the Arabs, or khorah of the Indians. In Arabia it is also called d'atil aül, a name corresponding with the leontiasis of the Greeks [1].

The distemper never appears among such of the Turks as are rich enough to afford themselves fresh meat, rice, and pulse through the year; nor among those Greeks who inhabit the mountains, and whose food consists partly of milk, fruits, and herbs. For the course of an hundred years, during which the French have been settled in Candia, none of them have ever been attacked by the leprosy *."

* Letters on Greece.

CHAP. V.

GENERAL DISEASES.

DRACUNCULUS, OR GUINEA-WORM. CHIGRES.

DRACUNCULUS, vena medinensis, or Guinea-worm *, is not often met with upon the Windward Coast of Africa, but appears to be nearly confined to that part of it called the Gold Coast.

The inhabitants of the river Gambia, and they who live between that river and the Senegal, are said to be affected with the Guinea-worm, but at no other time than the dry season, when the water is bad. Moore mentions an instance of a woman who had, within two months, a worm a yard long extracted from each knee, and soon afterwards another from the ankle †. A slave trader in the Rio Nunez informed me

* History of Gambia.

† The frequent occurrence of the disease upon the coast of Guinea has occasioned this name to be applied to it. Kemmersamius, an old writer, says, it is very frequent at Del Mina, on the Gold Coast, and the adjacent country, and that the natives are more affected with it than the Germans who trade there. As something marvellous is expected from a foreign country, and, according to the old proverb, ex Africa semper aliquid novi, the same author adds, that those persons who only sail past these places feel an itching in their arms, legs, and thighs. Mangetus Bib. Chir.

that the inhabitants of the kingdom of Bouree, a country from which much gold is brought, and situated about four days journey from Teembo, towards Tombuctoo, are greatly troubled with the Guinea-worm, which he has often seen in the slaves brought from that country. It does not appear that the disease could have been there caused by drinking bad water, as he says the natives of Bouree take only the water of springs. Whites as well as blacks are affected with the dracunculus, though more frequently the latter, as they use fewer precautions against it. That this disease originates upon the Gold Coast, from the badness of the water seems probable from the worm being seldom found in those parts, where, to guard against it, they take the precaution of boiling the water they drink *. It is not equally frequent on all parts of the Gold Coast, but is most prevalent where they have the worst water. At Annamaboo the Guinea-worm is very often met with. Dr. Trotter, speaking of the bad water at Annamaboo, says, " This water was taken from a stagnant lake, and so full of animalcules, that when strained through a stone, and kept a few hours, it again

---

* Mr. Park says, the Guinea-worm is very common in certain places, especially at the *commencement* of the rainy season, and is attributed by the negroes to the badness of the water. " They allege," he observes, " that the people who drink from wells, are more subject to it than those who drink from streams. To the same cause they attribute the swelling of the glands of the neck, (goitres) which are very common in some parts of Bambarra."

exhibited the like number of living atoms. It
had likewise the effect of producing the Guinea-worm among the negroes first purchased,
who had no signs of it till living on this water for some months *." At Cape Coast the
Guinea-worm is less frequent than at the above-
mentioned place, and Dix Cove is least of all
affected with it. At Whidah, where they have
good water, this complaint is not known, but
at Akra †, which is only sixty miles from thence,
it is very common. Loefler ‡ observes, that
" this worm is most prevalent in the English
and Dutch settlements on the coast of Africa."
He adds, " out of two hundred and twenty slaves,
which were bought at Cape Mount, Cape Mezu-
rado, and Cape La Hou, only one was affected
with Guinea-worm, which occurred in the great
toe. On the contrary, among sixty slaves which
were bought at St. George del Mina, a third part
laboured under this disease; and among six hundred slaves bought at Angola, not a single instance of it occurred." The Guinea-worm is also
unknown in the islands of Saint Thomas and
Prince. Barbot says, he was assured that the
natives inland, at the distance of forty or fifty
leagues from the sea coast, are unacquainted with
the Guinea-worm ; he further adds, that it is most

* Observations on the Scurvy.
† Isert Reise nach. Guinea.
‡ Chirurgische Wahrnehmungen. in Archiv. der Pract. Arz-
ney kunst.

frequent about Kormantyn and Apam, and that
Akra * is most free from it. The Guinea-worm
is little known in the West India Islands, except
among slaves lately imported from Africa. Dr.
Rouppe †, however, asserts, that it is very frequent in the Dutch island of Curacoa, where he
wishes to prove that it is contagious, and that
sailors become frequently affected by being " connected with Europeans and Negroes who have
the disorder." " That it is contagious," he adds,
" is very evident, as it never is in a house without
infecting the whole family, because these little
animals, and their seed, are carried about in the
bodies of the living from place to place, and communicated from one to the other. Some of the
inhabitants of this island, people of credit, have
told me, that this disorder is not of very long
standing amongst them, and that it was brought
there by the negroes who came from Guinea.
Dr. Chisholm also, in his Essay on the Malignant
Pestilential Fever of the West Indies, classes this
disease among the *epidemics* of the island of Grenada. Upon this subject, he observes in a note,
" it will appear singular to the European reader,
that the dracunculus, or Guinea-worm, should be
classed among the epidemics of Grenada; but,
however strange it may seem, it is nevertheless

* It is observed by an old writer, that those who touch at
Mouree, on the Gold Coast, are sooner affected with this disease than those who visit Akra. Dapper Description de l'A-
frique.

† On the Diseases of Seamen.

fully established by innumerable facts. One very extraordinary instance will suffice to show the propriety of considering this disease as one of the epidemics of the dry season. On the estates of Edmund Thornton, Esq. situated in the district of St. George's Parish, called Point Saline, already described, and at the farthest extremity of it, the negroes are attacked regularly every year, about the beginning of November, with symptoms of the Guinea-worm. In the month of January, the disease spreads throughout the greatest part of the gang, and in the month of March it entirely disappears; and they continue exempted from it till the following November. The cause of this singular disease on the estates I have mentioned, seems to be confined to the water of some wells, which have been dug in the substance called tuf, (a soft rocky substance, probably of volcanic origin, and perhaps the tuffa of the Italians) of which the whole gang drink, there being no springs or rivulets in the district, and unfortunately no cisterns to collect and preserve the rain water. This has been rendered evident by what has happened on some neighbouring estates, the negroes of which, till of late, were as subject to this distressing complaint as those belonging to Mr. Thornton. The wells were filled up, cisterns built, or wells dug in places not subject to the influence of the flow and ebb of the tide, and at the return of the usual period of the appearance of the Guinea-worm, nothing of the kind happened. They

have ever since (three years now) continued exempted from the disease. In the water which
contains the embryos of the dracunculi, the
naked eye distinguishes innumerable animalcules,
darting in every direction with astonishing force
and rapidity ; these, on being subjected to examination in a small microscope, exhibit a very
extraordinary figure, differing from any animalcules hitherto described." The curious appearance of these animalcules has induced many
writers to believe that they are changed into the
Guinea-worm when received into the stomach ;
but there is greater reason to believe that they
are hatched from the ova of musquitos. They
are seen in myriads in rain water, when permitted to stagnate, and are found in abundance in the rain water tubs at Free Town,
where the Guinea-worm has never occurred.
Mr. Bruce says, " the worm known to the Arabian physicians, under the name of vena medinensis, and by the natives called *pharoum*, or
Pharoah's worm, is so named from the city of
Medina, where Mahomet was buried, and which
is distant from the sea about three days journey.
They believe that this malady, as well as the
small pox, and several others, were not known
before the time of that impostor. Aga Thareide,
the Gnidian, has, however, spoken of it several
centuries before the Christian æra, as an endemial disorder on the coasts of the Red Sea. It
is common also in Arabia the Happy, Arabia the
Desert, on the coasts of the Persian Gulph, and

in the peninsula of India. It prevails likewise on the coasts of Africa, and in all the low and burnt border of land which surrounds that part of the world, from the ocean to the Mediterranean. It extends to the interior part of the country, to Arfour, Sallee, Bargina in Nubia, and even as far as to Egypt."

" In all the countries of Asia and Africa, which I have already named, the inhabitants drink stagnated water, because the tropical rains which fall from the mountains are collected in the plains among the sands. Bassora, and the coasts of Persia, are, indeed, on this side of the tropic, but the inhabitants have nothing to drink except water of that kind, which they find among the sand. The people in the mountainous parts, near those countries which I have mentioned, are not acquainted with this worm, neither is it known in Abyssinia, and the elevated part of Arabia the Happy, but those who descend from thence to live on the borders of the sea, where the country is dry and sandy, as is the case with Nubia, are much troubled with it *."

It is said that at Bokhara, the present capital of Usbec Tartary, one hundred and thirty-eight miles southwest of Samarcand, the ancient capital of that country, the inhabitants are much subject to the Guinea-worm, owing to the bad water they drink.

According to Niebuhr, this worm occurs very

* Travels in Abyssinia.

frequently in Yemen, in the peninsula of India, and at Gambroon, or Bender Abbas, in Persia. It is called at Loheia, ark ; and at Haleb (Aleppo) ark el insil. A merchant of Mecca, whom he met with at Bombay, called it farentit ; and at Abuschähr, near the Persian gulf, it is called peju and naru, though he apprehends the three last words may not be Arabic, but Persian or Indian. They attribute it in these countries to drinking bad water, for which reason many of the Arabs filter, through linen, the water whose qualities they are not well acquainted with.

The dracunculi are said by Professor Pallas to be found no where more abundantly than in Russia ; and the celebrated Weikard found them in great numbers in the canals of Petersburg, and in the river Neva. There is a disease in Russia called wolosaz, with which the Moors are affected, and which has been called the *hair disease*, because they imagine that hair cut off, and thrown into water, is changed into worms, which insinuate themselves into the bodies of those who bathe there, and thus produce ulcers. Gmelin saw a worm of this kind, which was about six inches long, as small as a hair, and was probably a gordius. In the lakes and marshes in Siberia, especially between the rivers Irtisch and Obi, the gordius is found in abundance. It is said also to abound in the waters of the Swedish province of West Gothland *.

* Finke versuch einer algemein. Medic. Pract. Geographie.

The opinions of authors have varied considerably respecting the nature of the dracunculus;
some have supposed it to be merely a vein, and
hence it received the name it bears among the
Arabian writers; others imagined it to be a
nerve or tendon *; and several of the moderns,
among whom was the celebrated Ambrose Parè,
thought that it consisted only of coagulated pus,
an opinion which scarce requires to be formally
contradicted. The most just, and generally received opinion at present is, that it is a real animal. As such it is thus accurately described by Sauvages, " vere vermis est——rostello barbato, pi-
lis tenuissimis, cum puncto atri coloris, & oris ves-
tigio quodam: in cauda etiam punctum foraminis
est instar ani—patria est terra æstuosa, tor-
rens, cœlum intemperatum, solum arenosum, ste-
rile salsum, aqua destitutum, ubi aqua ex cisternis
hausta, eaque sæpe impura, verminosa bibitur."
Nos. Meth. Bajon also observes, " it is a real
worm, in which irritability and sensibility are
very evident. When divided transversely, it appears to consist of five or six pretty strong
threads, united by means of a very fat cellular
texture, like a strong glue †." Many instances
are also recorded wherein the worm was observed
to move about briskly, after having been ex-

* In quodam Arabiæ loco, ut aiunt, in tibiis hominum dracunculi vocati nascuntur, nervosa natura, colore, crassitudineque
lumbricis similes. Multos sanè audivi, qui sese vidisse eos di-
cerent; ipse vero nunquam vidi, neque de ortu, neque de essentia
ipsorum quidquam exacte conjicere possum." Galen de Locis
affectis, lib. vi. c. 3.

† Nachrichten zur Geschichte von Cayenne.

tracted from the body, and put into a vessel full of warm water.

Different opinions are likewise entertained respecting the mode in which this worm is received into the body, each of which has difficulties not easily solved.——If, because the disease is almost exclusively found in those countries where the water is bad, it be supposed that the worm is received into the stomach with the drink, either in the oviform or animalcular state, it may be objected, that every person who makes use of this water in its pure or raw state is not affected with the disease. Moreover, it has never been found in animals, whether in a wild or domestic state, though drinking of the same kind of water. The Guinea-worm is rarely found in deep seated muscular parts, a circumstance which militates against this opinion ; and there is, I believe, no instance on record of its having been observed in any of the abdominal viscera.

If, on the contrary, from its more frequent occurrence in the inferior extremities, than in other parts of the body, and from its superficial situation, it be supposed to be insinuated by puncture through the integuments, either as an egg or animalcule, this implies such a degree of defective instinct, as is seldom or never observed in animated nature. In other instances we find the parent insect deposit its ova in situations where the young, when hatched, can not only procure food, but have also a retreat secured, in which they may undergo a further change. Astruc

supposes that the Guinea-worm would change
into a fly, or butter-fly, and adduces in support
of this opinion, the worms found in the amyg-
dalæ of stags, in the nostrils of sheep, and upon
the backs of oxen, which afterwards leave these
situations, and are changed into flies. But here
the analogy fails, for the Guinea-worm, whether
it leave its nidus to enter into the chrysalis state,
or as a perfect animal, to propagate its species,
almost certainly dies.

Mr. Bruce is of opinion, that the guinea-worm
is not produced from the ova deposited in stagnant water, taken into the stomach and hatched
there ; but thinks he has discovered the insect by
which it is produced. " It resembles," he says,
" a bug; has its two fore feet armed with claws,
and its trunk with a kind of forceps, for the purpose of tearing and wounding. This insect is
found in stagnant water ; it attaches itself to the
legs and arms, which are the parts of the body
most usually naked in warm climates and sel-
domest washed, and there deposes its eggs in the
cellular tissue, until they are hatched by the
warmth of spring." There is reason to think
this opinion ill founded, for we find, in general,
some degree of proportion exist between the
young and the animal which gives it birth ; but
in the present instance, the disproportion between
an insect the size of a bug and a worm a yard
long is too striking to pass unnoticed.

The dracunculus is always situated in the cellular substance, between the skin and the mus-

cles, most frequently of the feet and legs ; but it is sometimes met with in the arms, hands, thighs, body, and even in the head. The worm is generally about the thickness of a crow's quill or a piece of cat-gut, of a white or bluish colour, and shining like a tendon. It is in general from a foot to three or four feet in length.

It sometimes happens that there is more than one worm in the body at the same time. Rhazes* mentions an instance of a person who was cured after having forty of these worms in his body : Avicenna also asserts, that though the patient have forty or fifty worms in his body at one time, he may be cured ; which shews that the disease, when treated with care, is not fatal, and seldom even dangerous.

The situation of the dracunculus is sometimes so superficial that its convolutions may be distinctly perceived underneath the integuments. In such cases, if an incision be made over the middle of the worm, it may frequently be extracted double : where this cannot be done, the worm must be divided, and the ends be drawn out separately, as different worms †. A curious case is related by Bajon, of a negro girl, about six or seven years of age, who had one of these worms in her eye. It was situated between the tunica albuginea and sclerotica, being about two inches long, and not thicker than a common thread :

---

* Friend Hist. Medic. p. 149.
† Loefler Chirurgische wahrnehmungen.

it moved very briskly, and in a serpentine direction about the eye. The patient experienced no pain from the motion of the worm, nor was the eye affected in its appearance, though it was constantly weeping. He extracted the worm by seizing it in the middle with a pair of forceps, and drawing it double through a small opening made with a lancet in the tunica adnata. The patient was cured in twenty-four hours. A similar instance occurred to him in another negro girl, somewhat elder than the last : the eye was inflamed and painful, and in it he discovered a worm rather larger than the one before mentioned, which moved in the same manner round the globe of the eye. He was not permitted to extract it, as in the former case; nor did he learn how the case terminated *. In the Edinburgh Medical Essays, (vol. v.) a case is related, in which, from five or six ulcers on the legs, in the space of eight weeks, were extracted " thirty yards of the dracunculus, after which the ulcers healed, and cicatrised with no trouble:" one of these worms was three yards and a half in length. When the animal has reached a certain size, it begins to excite some degree of disturbance and uneasiness in that part where the head is nearest to the surface, generally where a bone is least covered with flesh. A slight degree of heat is felt in the part, succeeded by a small, hard, and inflamed tumor, resembling a common boil,

* Nachrichten zur Gesch. von Cayenne.

attended with much pain, and larger, or smaller, according to the size of the worm. These symptoms are for the most part preceded by a febrile attack, accompanied with rigors. The tumor gradually increases in size, becoming more pointed : the skin assumes a shining red colour, and is attenuated, a fluctuation being felt beneath it. At this period the disease has no other appearance than that of a boil, and it is only in those countries where it is endemial that they suspect it in its early state. Whenever the tumor bursts, the head of the worm shews itself like a black speck, and the disease is evident. As soon as a part of the leg begins to swell, and becomes painful, the natives of Africa endeavour to promote suppuration as quickly as possible : with this view, the inhabitants of El Mina apply a cataplasm of the leaves of the volkameria acuminata, beaten up with a few pods of red pepper, which is repeated every day until the skin breaks. About Akra the natives bruise the leaves of the cissus quadrangularis, which they apply every day to the tumefied part. The next point of practice is the same in every nation where this disease exists, and was first described by Leonidas, who was a surgeon at Alexandria, about the end of the fifth century *. As soon as the

---

* De Brachiorum ac Crurum Dracunculis. Leonidæ, cap. lxxxv. Qui appellantur dracunculi lumbricis similes sunt, & aliquando magni, aliquando parvi reperiuntur, frequentius quidem in cruribus, quandoque vero & in musculosis brachiorum partibus consistentes. Nascuntur autem hi in Æthiopia ac India, in pueris præci-

head of the worm appears, it is laid hold of, and
gently rolled around a piece of stick until the patient feel a little pain, when they desist from
winding, and cover the wound with a soft leaf
or piece of plaster. The same operation is repeated every day with great caution, until the
whole be extracted. If by too much haste or
violence in winding it, the worm be broken, and
the end cannot be again recovered, the part in-
flames, and becomes intolerably painful; an attack of fever - supervenes, frequently attended
with a train of alarming symptoms, until suppuration again take place, and the end of the worm

pue, estque ipsorum generatio non dissimilis lumbricis latis ventris.
Sub cute enim moventur nihil molestiæ afferentes, verum temporis
progressu circa dracunculi extremitatem locus suppuratur, &
cutis aperitur, ac dracunculi caput exeritur. Quod si dracunculus attrahatur vehementem dolorem inducit, præsertim si nimia
tractus violentia fuerit ruptus: nam quod relinquitur, molestis-
simos dolores infert. Proinde ut ne recurrat animal, valido filö
brachium constringere oportet, & quotidie hoc moliri, ut dracunculus paulatim progrediens constrictione quidem intercludatur,
nequaquam autem abrumpatur. Locus item aqua mulsa, & oleo
in quo absinthium aut abrotonum coctum est, aut alio quodam
ex his quæ ad alvi lumbricos descripsimus, irrigandus est. Omnia tamen acria vitanda, propter periculum inflammationis. Ca-
taplasmata quoque laxatoria ac suppuratoria e farinis cum aqua
mulsa & oleo præparata adhibeantur. Quod si dracunculus sponte
progrediens facile extrahi poterit, nihil amplius faciendum est.
Sin ad suppurationem vertetur, a cataplasmatis, & aquæ mulsæ ac
olei rigatione non est discedendum. Nos vero emplastrum e
baccis lauri, post cataplasmatum ablationem, imponere solemus,
facta vero suppuratione, cutis per longitudinem dissecetur, &
dracunculus denudatus auferatur, & cutis linamentis inditis dis-
paretur, & reliqua curatio suppuratoria adhibeatur, ita ut ani-
mali suppurato & extracto, ulcus incarnetur & ad cicatricem per-
ducatur. Aetii Tetrabil. 4. s. 2.

be protruded. Nothing further is practised during the extraction of the worm than to plunge the limb into cold water occasionally, which is the most effectual means of relieving the pain, but never applied until the suppurative process be completed. When the worm is wholly extracted, the wound generally heals without further trouble : but the repeated occurrence of this disease may perhaps occasion the ulcerated legs so frequently seen upon the Gold Coast.

The general health is not affected by the dracunculi, however numerous. Several remedies are recommended to promote their quicker expulsion. Professor Gmelin recommends a solution of corrosive sublimate in brandy, given internally in the usual dose. This remedy, however, is said by Loefler * to have had no good effect in the cases in which he used it ; on the contrary, the slaves lost their appetites, becoming lean and dejected. From other internal remedies he experienced as little benefit, and none from the use of aloes, which has been particularly recommended. Of external applications, he found mercurial frictions rather prejudicial, inasmuch as they increased the tumor, and therefore rendered the extraction of the worm less easy. He perceived most benefit from rubbing the part with volatile liniment, which dispersed the tumor, and diminished the pain.

* Chirurgische Wahrnehmungen.

Another very celebrated remedy consists of
bruised garlic, flour of mustard, black pepper,
flowers of sulphur, each one ounce, mixed in a
quart of spirits ; of this a wine glass full is to be
taken every other morning for nine times. According to Dr. Bancroft, the most successful mode
of treating this disease is to apply a cataplasm of
onions and bread boiled in milk to the swelling,
and when the head of the worm appears to secure
it by a piece of cotton, without making any attempt to extract the body. At the same time he
orders *half a gill* of the abovementioned mixture
(omitting the flour of mustard) to be drank morning and evening, by which means, in a day or two,
he adds, the worm will be found coiled up under
the poultice. The same author mentions another
kind of worm found in Guiana, resembling a bean,
but more slender and pointed, which is bred in
the muddy stagnant waters in the woods, and in-
serts itself into the flesh, chiefly about the ankles:
when extracted it leaves a sinuous callous ulcer,
which is difficultly cured *.

How long the Guinea-worm may lie concealed
in the body is not certainly known, but it frequently remains several months there without
exciting the smallest degree of pain, or raising
any suspicion of its presence. Dr. Isert, whilst
in the island of Martinico, *eight* months after his
return from Africa, having fatigued himself very

* History of Guiana, 389

much with walking, was affected with a considerable swelling of his left leg. He could attribute this to no particular cause. The swelling continued for thirty-six hours, and then disappeared. A fortnight afterwards, having walked the whole day, and waded much in the water, he observed upon the same foot which had swelled before, a small vesicle, and on opening it, was surprised to find a gordius medinensis; this he attempted to draw out, but could only obtain a few inches on account of the excessive pain occasioned by the trial. Hence also, probably, was excited a degree of symptomatic fever, which continued the whole night. After this he treated the worm in a very simple manner, winding it every day upon a roll of linen, and covering the whole with a cloth, which enabled him to continue his usual walks. He attributed the speediness of the cure, which was completed in eight days, though in Africa it usually takes up some months, to his using so much exercise, and wading at the same time in the water. The worm was one of the largest he had seen : it measured two ells in length, and was of the thickness of a straw *.

A similar instance is noticed by Dr. Rouppe, " in a Dutch man of war, which came from Curacoa to Holland, before she went to the Mediterranean. Neither in Holland, nor in the island, nor in her whole voyage, did any symptom of these worms appear ; but after a short stay in the

* Reise nach Guinea.

Mediterranean, above a third part of the crew
was confined to their hammocks by them, nor
were the sailors only troubled with them, but the
officers likewise." Niebuhr also relates, that Mr.
Cramer perceived four of these worms in his feet,
and one in his hand, more than five months from
the time of leaving Arabia; but as he lived only
ten or twelve days after the discovery, none of them
had time to come out. A remarkable instance
is related of a person at Rochelle, in France, who
had never been in Africa, but was affected with
a Guinea-worm, owing to his having drank some
water on board a ship, which had been brought
from the coast of Guinea *. " One of our sailors, says Loefler, who had slept several nights
on shore in Africa, was affected, whilst in England, a year afterwards, with a Guinea-worm in
one of his legs; it was broken in the extraction,
and produced suppuration, and several indurated
tumors. By means of incisions and emollient
cataplasms the patient was freed from every symptom of the disease †."

This disease occurred in a more severe manner
to Mr. Bruce, upon his return from Abyssinia,
which he thus describes: " I was not affected
with this malady in Arabia, though I resided
there some time in the maritime regions; nor do
I think that I contracted it in Abyssinia. I am

* See Professor Finke's elaborate and interesting work, Versuch einer allgemein. medicin. praktisch. Geographie, vol. ii.
p. 53.

† Chirurgische wahrnehmungen.

rather of opinion, that it began when I was crossing the desert of Nubia, and the country of the Funges. On the first of April, *five months* after my departure from Nubia, I felt an itching above the thick part of my leg, and having scratched it a little, it began to swell, as if stung by a gnat, and the worm appeared then to be perfectly white. Next morning, this small wound was a little inflamed. I felt neither pain nor itching from it, and the worm made no attempt to come forth. From this period to the second of May, I applied nothing to the sore, which was very moist by an abundant discharge of a watery humour.

I embarked then to return to Europe, and having passed great part of the night on deck, when I attempted to retire, I found my knee so stiff, that I could not walk. I undressed myself, and observed upon the rotula a tumor of the size of an egg, which had scarcely any inflammation, but was exceedingly painful. By the advice of some Arabs, I applied a cataplasm of lintseed, and after a night passed in the greatest agony, about an inch and a half of the worm came out, of a livid transparent colour, but different from what it had appeared to be at first. During the two following days, it continued to come out about an inch every day. The swelling and pain increased every moment, in such a manner, that though the wound was in the interior part of the calf of the leg, four inches below the knee, the thigh, leg, and foot were so much swelled that I could not support the bed clothes without crying out through pain. The inflammation was not considerable any where but around the sore, which was of a deep red colour, and discharged a quantity of matter.

After four days, the surgeon of the ship broke the worm, by taking off the cataplasm of lint-seed too hastily, and that night the whole leg, from the rotula to the heel, swelled so much that it all appeared to be of the same thickness. In this painful situation I continued for fifty-eight days. After using several remedies, and cataplasms of emollient herbs, without any success, and after suffering a great deal, I observed a part of the tumor a little more elevated than the rest. Having pressed it with my finger, it discharged about three ounces of matter, and continuing to press my leg in the like manner with my fingers, at certain intervals, the rest of the worm came out; the wound closed the same night; the pain decreased, and no more swelling appeared, but at the knee. Several tumors were observed afterwards below the rotula, and I apprehended that they would form there a collection of matter, but in a short time they disappeared, and my knee recovered its strength, though very slowly." This worm was about two feet in length. Mr. Bruce says, the Banians, in the East Indies, are the only people who have the art of making this worm come forth quickly of itself. He has seen them apply cataplasms of certain leaves to those who were attacked with this disorder, and has observed the next morning the whole worm under the cataplasm, while the leg was very little affected. These leaves are said to grow only on the coast of Malabar, and the knowledge of them is carefully concealed.

The following case of Guinea-worm which occurred in the person of a surgeon in the East India company's service, though defective in not pointing out where the disease was acquired, and in some other particulars, contains much curious information.*

" About the end of November, 1791, I perceived an unusual stiffness and soreness in the inferior part of the gastrocnemii muscles of the right leg, at that part where the tendons of both gastrocnemii unite to form the tendo achillis. This soreness was never acute, consequently did not occasion particular inconvenience, or prevent me from walking. Several days afterwards I observed a swelling in the part; but this was not attended by an increase of pain, nor discoloration. A few days after the occurrence of the swelling, a small reddish-coloured pustule, with a black point in the middle, appeared on the inside of the leg, about an inch above the malleolus internus, on the fleshy part of the leg, and behind the tibia. This pustule appeared to contain a watery fluid. At the same time, I felt very distinctly, under the skin, a round firm substance, and was able

* Ed. Med. Commentaries, Dec. 1, vol. viii.

to trace the animal with my finger to a consider
able distance, extending in convolutions obliquely
towards the posterior and upper part of the leg.
Though the disease was *now* evident, yet I did
not think it necessary to use any remedies with
a view to expedite the animal's progress; nor,
indeed, was I acquainted with any medicine or
application which could produce that effect. I
concluded that he would work his way out, and
that it would be most prudent to leave him un-
molested; but, on the night of the 17th December, a few days after the appearance of the
pustule, though I went to bed otherwise in perfect health, I awoke, at two in the morning, with
a sensation of intolerable itching over the whole
surface of the body. This sensation was so extremely urgent, that I could not refrain from
scratching violently. Soon afterwards, I felt an
excessive heat and pricking in my face. On
looking in a glass, I remarked a redness and flush-
ing over my face, and the muscles of the face
were swelled and convulsed. On those parts of
my skin, where I felt the itching, I could discover
with my finger, a thickening, as it were, of the
skin; it felt as if full of hard bumps. While puz-
zled to account for these symptoms, which I had
never seen, nor read, nor heard of, I was attacked
with excruciating pain in my belly, accompanied
by violent retching, vomiting, and loose stools.
A little bile and acid matter were rejected, by
vomiting. But as very little bile, notwithstanding the violent retching, was brought up, or

passed downwards, these symptoms could not have been occasioned by an unusual quantity or acrimony of that fluid. The vomiting, as nearly as I can guess, continued with very little intermission above half an hour, during the whole of which time the pain continued with unabated severity. These symptoms were succeeded by violent rigors, which continued for some hours, and resembled the cold stage of the paroxysm of an intermittent unusually severe. When the vomiting ceased, I went to bed, and was well covered with blankets. The sensation of cold gradually abated, and I fell asleep. The coldness and shivering were not followed by any preternatural degree of heat of which I was sensible; but when I awoke in the morning, I felt a moisture on my feet. In the course of the night, the pustule had burst, and a white firm substance appeared in the spot which the pustule had occupied, but so deep that it could not be laid hold of. The animal had changed his situation during the preceding night, and had buried himself very deeply among the muscles. He had effected this so completely, that though I felt him with my finger to a great extent on the 17th, yet, on the morning of the 18th, there was not the smallest portion perceptible; nor could I discover the least trace, on the strictest examination. I felt no inconvenience from the attack, which I have described, on the following day, except a little weakness; nor had I afterwards any return of these distressing symptoms. On the night of the 18th, a considerable inflammation appeared surrounding the ankle, and I found it necessary, on the 19th, to refrain from walking, and to confine myself to a horizontal position. On the 22d, I drew a small thread across the surface of the sore, so as to touch the extremity of the animal, which felt hard, and firmly fixed in the flesh. In consequence of this irritation, he threw up a considerable quantity of a watery fluid. Some time after this, he entirely disappeared, and the inflammation abated. A troublesome sore remained, with a bloody ichorous discharge, which continued until the beginning of February, 1792. It then healed, except a small point. At this time the animal made his appearance, and I was enabled to secure him with a thread. He was wrapped round a small bit of stick, and pulled twice a day, in the common manner. At the expiration of twenty days, the extraction was completed.

The animal was upwards of two yards in length, and of the thickness of a crow quill. After the half was extracted, he gradually diminished in size. I found that his progress was quickened by the application of the aloe leaf, as hot as it could be borne, to that part of the leg which was hard, swelled, and painful. The same effect was produced by hard friction."

This complaint, according to Ulloa, occurs also in South America, but not so frequently " as the

leprosy, itch, and herpes;" it is there called co-
brilla, or little snake, which they suppose has
insinuated itself beneath the skin. " The external
indications of it are, a round, inflamed tumor,
of the thickness of a quarter of an inch, attended
with a slight pain, but not vehement, and a numb-
ness of the part, which often terminates in a mortification." The natives first examine where, according to their phrase, the head is, to which
they apply a small suppurative plaister, and
gently foment the whole tumor with oil. The
next day the skin under the plaister is found divided, and through the orifice appears a kind of
white fibre, about the size of a coarse sewing
thread, and this, according to them, is the cobril-
la's head, which they carefully fasten to a thread
of silk, and wind the other end of it about a card,
rolled up like a cylinder. The fomentation with
oil is continued, and the worm is rolled round
the cylinder every day, until the whole be extracted*.

There is a complaint with which negroes in the
West Indies are frequently affected, and which
bears a faint resemblance to the last, in being
produced by an insect burrowing under the skin :
when properly treated it is of no importance,
but when neglected it frequently endangers the
loss of toes and feet. This insect is called chigre †,

* Ulloa's Voyage to South America, i. 46.
† Malis Americana Sauvagesii. It is said to disappear during
the rainy season, at which time the negroes are free from them.

pulex penetrans; it is a very small black insect,
somewhat resembling a flea, but much smaller.
It is found about the hearths of houses which
are ill swept and dirty, and chiefly affects
those who go with naked feet, and are not very
cleanly. This insect generally insinuates itself
under the skin between the toes, where it forms
to itself a small bag, like an hydatid, about the
size of a pea, in which it deposits its innumerable
ova. The cure consists in extracting this bag
whole by means of a sharp pointed instrument,
which is done by the negro women with great
dexterity. If this bag be carelessly burst, each
ovum, when hatched, forms for itself a fresh bag
or nidus. An uncomfortable degree of itching
is the only symptom which indicates the early
state of the disease. Ligon describes this curious
insect as " not much unlike a louse, but no bigger
than a mite that breeds in cheese, his colour
blewish: an Indian has laid one of them on a
sheet of white paper, and with my spectacles on
I could hardly discern him;——this vermine
will get through your stocken, and in a pore of
your skinne, in some part of your feet, commonly
under the nayl of your toes, and there make a
habitation to lay his offspring, as bigge as a small
tare, or the bagge of a bee, which will cause you
to go very lame, and put you to much smarting
paine,

" The Indian (negro) women have the best skill
to take them out, which they do by putting in

a small poynted pinne or needle, at the hole where he came in, and winding the poynt about the bagge, loosen him from the flesh, and so take him out.——I have had tenne taken out of my feet in a morning, by the most unfortunate *Yarico,* an Indian woman *."

* Ligon was at Barbadoes in the year 1647.

CHAP. VI.

GENERAL DISEASES.

ENLARGEMENT OF THE SCROTUM. ENLARGEMENT OF
THE LEGS. GOUT. RHEUMATISM. PLEURISY.
DISEASED LIVER. SCROPHULA. PHTHISIS. ANO-
REXIA. SPITTING OF BLOOD.

IT is not uncommon to meet with persons on
the coast labouring under a prodigious EN-
LARGEMENT OF THE SCROTUM, which to those unacquainted with medicine, gives the idea of an im-
mensely large rupture, and has occasioned travellers to assert that the Africans are very liable
to be affected with ruptures. It is called by the
Bulloms, kok ; by the Timmanees, ka-rot ; and by
the Soosoos, key-key. Upon the Gold Coast this
disease, sarcoma scrotale is very frequent, and about
El Mina it is called dekapatrosè, where it is supposed to be occasioned by drinking palm wine to
excess. This opinion, though grounded only on
popular prejudice, appears strengthened by the
complaint being most prevalent where palm wine
abounds most. The Bagoes, a nation which in-
habits the south shore of the Rio Nunez and Ca-
patches, where the palm tree grows in great plenty,
are more subject to this complaint than the Nalloes, who live on the north side of the same river,
and have not so many of the palm trees among

them. It must however be remarked that the Bagoes labour under a scarcity of good water, especially during the dry season, the ground being very low and swampy, and the water brackish : the Nalloes, on the contrary, have an abundance of good water. It is therefore more probable that this complaint originates from the bad quality of the water, as it occurs sometimes among the Mahommedans, who religiously abstain from palm wine. I have seen three instances of the disease, two of which were old men, apparently near fifty years of age : in neither of them could the tumor weigh less than forty or fifty pounds. When the patients sat upon the ground, the tumor rested upon a cotton cloth, which served also to support the troublesome weight when they moved. The complaint had been in both cases of many years standing, and had encreased very gradually, indeed almost imperceptibly. It was attributed to drinking too freely of palm wine. The third instance occurred in a handsome young man, about twenty-two years of age, tall, and remarkably well formed ; the disease had advanced in him more rapidly than usual, as he had been affected with it only four years. The tumor reached nearly as low as his knees, when he stood erect, and might probably weigh twenty pounds. The penis was entirely concealed in the skin of the scrotum, as in a large hydrocele. The testes were distinctly to be felt at the upper part of the tumor, pressed close to the penis, and were of the natural size. The spermatic cord was neither enlarged nor painful. The lower part of the tumor had acquired an almost cartilaginous hardness, and the surface was deeply furrowed : on the sides, the integuments were apparently much thickened, and there seemed to be an obscure degree of fluctuation within. This induced me to push in a trocar, which he readily allowed, but nothing issued except a few drops of blood. He experienced no pain from the complaint, unless after it had hung down for a length of time, without its usual support, when he felt some uneasiness from its weight.

This disease is said to be endemic among the inhabitants of Bambarra, and among the Mandingos in the kingdom of Barra. Dr. Schotte* observed the same complaint in a negro at Senegal, about fifty years of age : the scrotum weighed at least half a hundred weight; it measured eighteen inches in diameter, and two feet and a half in length. The swelling had begun twenty-five years before, by an almost imperceptible enlargement of the testicles, devoid of pain. In Galam the rich inhabitants are peculiarly subject to this disease; and when they ride on horseback, the tumor is placed in a wooden case fixed to the fore part of the saddle.

The sarcoma scroti is supposed generally to be hereditary ; and is referred to the great quantity of pepper which is used in seasoning their food.

* Philos. Trans. vol. lxxii.

diment along the whole coast; but if the disease originated from this cause, the instances of it ought to be much more numerous *.

Upon the Gold Coast prodigious ENLARGEMENTS OF THE LEGS are often met with, which the natives attribute to the same cause as the last complaint, the immoderate use of palm wine; some of them being in the habit of drinking, upon an average, two gallons of this wine a day. The disease is frequent among the Bagoes, much less so among the Nalloes, and is said to be totally unknown among the Mandingos and Foolas. In the neighbourhood of El Mina, it is called appakookooa; the Bulloms call it oo-beng oo-hin-tay; the Timmanees, kat-tuk ka-buóy-a. They pay scarcely any attention to this complaint, as it does not affect the general health, and they use no remedies whatever. It generally affects but one leg, and seldom rises above the knee: the swelling is hard and firm, does not pit on pressure, and is entirely free from pain. It does not diminish the activity of the person, though it should render his leg as thick as his body. It is said to affect only those who have used palm wine immoderately, but it is more probably caused by the stagnant water which they are obliged to use.

This complaint appears to be exactly the same as that which occurs at Cochin, a Dutch settlement in the East Indies †, upon the banks of a river, in a low situation, supplied with bad

* Baldinger Medicinische Bibliothek ii. band. 4 stuck.
† Observ. on the Dis. of the East Indies, &c.

water. This is supposed to cause the enormous swellings, to which the natives are subject, and which are called in India Cochin legs. Dr. Clark observes, no European becomes affected with this disease, however long he may have resided there. " The natives of Cochin," he adds, " are extremely healthy; neither is the bulk of their legs the least inconvenience to them. No preternatural weight is to be observed: they are strong bodied, and enjoy as much agility as if they were totally exempt from this unseemly deformity *."

Notwithstanding the excesses committed by the pagan nations of Africa in the use of spirituous liquors, and the incitement which they have to excessive venery from a plurality of wives, I have never heard of an instance of GOUT among them, nor is it probable that they are acquainted with the disease. The Mahommedans are greatly debilitated by their frequent application to aphrodisiacs, and seldom fail, when they meet with European surgeons, to ask them for provocatives, or, as they phrase it, medicines " to strengthen the back." This demand is oftener made by them, than by their neighbours who use rum. A similar enquiry, as travellers observe, is usual among the Turks and Arabs. Dr. Rush informs us, that he has heard of two or three instances of gout among the Indians of

---

* See " Observations on the Diseases which prevail in long voyages to hot countries," by J. Clark, M. D. to whom we are indebted for an improved practice in the fevers of tropical climates.

North America, but only among those who had
learned the use of rum from the white people.
It does not appear how drinking of rum can
occasion gout, otherwise than by the general debility it induces. Dr. Rush observes, that the
reason why the gout does not appear more frequently among the class of people who use the
greatest quantity of rum in our own country
is, that " the effects of this liquor upon those en-
feebled people are too sudden and violent to
admit of their being thrown upon the extremities,
as we know them to be among the Indians ; they
appear only in visceral obstructions, and a com-
plicated train of chronic diseases. Thus putrid
miasmata are sometimes too strong to bring on
a fever, but produce instant debility and death."
It may, perhaps, give some support to this opinion, to observe that few of the inhabitants of
this part of Africa arrive at old age. They
turn old much sooner than Europeans, and
appear in a state of decrepitude when the
latter have scarcely reached their grand climac-
teric. Mr. Adanson makes the same remark :
" the negroes of Senegal," he observes, " are really
old at the age of forty-five, and oftentimes sooner :
and I remember to have heard the French inhabitants of Senegal say several times, that, according to the best of their observation, the negroes
of that country seldom lived to be older than
sixty *." From a want of fixed data, it is impossible for the most part to determine their ages

* Voyage to Senegal.

with any degree of precision. One instance only of longevity can be given with any degree of accuracy; this was in a person named Addoo, of considerable consequence, who resided in the river Sherbro, and who remembered, when a boy about fifteen years of age, to have been in the island of Barbadoes. This occurred during the reign of Queen Anne, or, as he expressed it, " when the king of England was a woman ;" consequently he must have been (in 1796) near one hundred years of age. He is still alive.

In a climate so intensely hot as that of Africa, it might be supposed that the natives would enjoy an immunity from the racking pains of RHEU-MATISM, which is by no means the case. They bring on these pains through the incautious manner in which they check perspiration, by throwing themselves upon the ground, and sleeping, after being fatigued by violent exertions in dancing, &c. Not unfrequently they sleep all night in the open air, especially during moon-light, exposed to the chilling dews which fall, and covered only with a thin cotton cloth. The pernicious effects of dew have already been noticed, although popular prejudice has referred them rather to the action of the moon's beams, it having been said, though without foundation, that animal substances, exposed to the light of the moon, very speedily corrupt. This appears to have been a very general error among the vulgar of all nations, except perhaps the Africans, who do not ascribe to the moon any influence on the human body.

Their favourite mode of cure for rheuma-

tism is by exciting a very copious and general
perspiration : with this view the earth-floor of
a hut is made very hot by live coals, and when
these are swept off, the floor is covered thickly
with the leaves of amelliky, nauclea sambucina,
previously sprinkled with water : upon these
are laid a mat and a cotton cloth for the patient
to recline on, and he is carefully covered up
with cloths, to promote the sweat. Professor
Finke, in his learned work (Versuch einer allge-
meinen medicinisch practischen Geographie) observes, that the best physicians are to be found
at Cape la Hou, whither they come from the
country of Saku. In several chronic diseases,
especially in rheumatism, they practise a curious
operation, that of exciting an artificial emphy-
sema, of which Gallandat * was an eye-witness.
When they find that the remedies employed have
no effect upon the disease, they make, with a
sharp instrument, an incision upon one or both
of the patient's legs, through the skin into
the cellular membrane. Into this wound they
introduce a hollow reed, or the stem of a pipe,
and blow as much air as they think necessary, or as the patient can support. The wound
is then covered with a piece of strongly adhesive
plaister, and a mixture composed of pepper, lime
juice, brandy, and certain herbs, is administered to
the patient. He is next ordered to run as vio-

* Abhandl. aus der Naturgeschichte, prakt. Arzneyk. hind
Chirurgie ; aus den schriften der Haarlemer, u. s. f. gezogen.
2 ter band.

lently as he can, and when overcome with fatigue, to betake himself to bed, where he remains a few days, being kept all the time in a profuse sweat. During this process a calibash full of the above-mentioned drink is administered every day, until the artificial tumor has disappeared, and the patient feels restored to health. The tumor generally begins to decline perceptibly about the third day, and on the 9th, 10th, or 11th days, it is no longer to be seen. Sometimes this operation is repeated in the same patient, of which Gallandat relates instances; he adds, that several negroes, whom he knew, assured him that they were cured by this means. In lumbago they drink a warm infusion of the root of a plant called by the Foolas gully-gully; by the Soosoos garangántang, and by the Bulloms ogboóg: it generally excites a copious perspiration.

Mr. Lucas, in his Communications to the African society, observes, " the diseases that are most frequent in Fezzan are those of the inflammatory and those of the putrid kind. The small pox is common among the inhabitants; violent headaches attack them in summer, and they are often afflicted with rheumatic pains. Their old women are their principal physicians. For pains of the head they prescribe cupping and bleeding; for pains in the limbs they send their patients to bathe in the hot lakes, which produce the trona, (mineral alkaly) and for obstináte head-achs and strains, and long continued stiffness in the muscles, they have recourse, like the horse doctors of

Europe, and the physicians of Barbary, to the application of a burning iron. The use of the strongest oils, and the most powerful herbs, is also frequent among them."

When the pain is confined to any particular spot, it is bathed with a decoction of the leaves and pods of the red pepper bush, or capsicum, used warm.

In pains of the neck, attended with stiffness and rigidity of the muscles, they apply as a cataplasm to the pained part a quantity of the leaves of the malip or plum tree, steeped in hot water: this is frequently repeated: and generally found very effectual.

When, in consequence of rheumatic pains, a stiffness of the joints remains, the leaves of a plant called by the Soosoos makootay, are bruised, soaked in hot water, and applied to the affected parts.

In deep seated pains of the limbs, contusions, or sprains, they apply the leaves of a plant called by the Soosoos karee, and by the Mandingos bannee: these are first bruised in a mortar, and heated over the fire before they are applied.

In pains of the side, either from rheumatic affection of the muscles, or pleurisy, they use the root of ayol bruised, and applied as a cataplasm; it contains a white juice, which is very acrid, and is capable of exciting blisters.

PLEURISY is a very rare disease among the natives, unless from external violence. An instance of peripneumony occurred to my knowledge, though I did not see the patient. It happened to a native greatly addicted to drinking spirits, and who had brought on the complaint by sleeping in the open air after intoxication. It terminated fatally in a few days, and to his friends very unexpectedly.

It has been remarked that black people brought to Europe are very liable to ABSCESS OF THE LIVER, a disease which occurs very rarely in Africa, and perhaps never idiopathically.

SCROPHULA, and its frequent concomitant, CONSUMPTION, are the diseases to which black people often fall victims in cold and variable climates: of the former complaint, only one or two instances occurred to me in Africa, and of the latter, as an idiopathic disease, I do not recollect to have seen a single case. An ingenious writer, speaking upon this subject, says, " our Indians are so tender, and habituated to a certain way of living, that they do not bear transplantation; for instance, the Spanish Indians, captivated in the St. Augustine war, anno 1702, and sold for slaves in New England, soon died consumptive *." Consumption is a very rare disease in the neighbourhood of Sierra Leone, but appears to be more common among the Foolas and Mandingos; it is called by the former nation do-eeróo, by the latter togo-sedaiya, or the " cough sickness;" the Susoos call it tago-myee, a word of the same import. In this disease, which they

---

* Gorden's Polit. Summary, i. p. 174.

look upon as incurable, they attend most to regimen, and especially prohibit the use of fat meat.
They do not suppose the disease to be infectious,
but·are of opinion that it often descends from
father to son.

At Teembo, as in all large towns, this disease
is very frequent. The place is indeed much more
unhealthy in proportion to the number of its
inhabitants, than other African cities. The cause
of this, as assigned to me by a Mandingo, was,
the many mixtures of different and very distant
people, with which the capital is always crowded.
Another cause probably is, the very confined
situation of Teembo. It has been supposed by
many, that a hot country is favourable to consumptive patients, but I have found the reverse
of this to be true. Among the Nova Scotia
settlers at Free Town, consumption occasionally
appeared, as a sequel of other diseases; and
in every instance, the fatal period occurred
much sooner than it would have done in England.

A very celebrated remedy in this disease is the
bark of a tree, called by the Foolas and Mandingos yay-goo ; and by the Soosoos cambay ;
it is a very powerful bitter : a decoction of the
bark is mixed with rice, of which they eat every
morning three handfuls.

In cases of COUGH, attended with a sensation of soreness at the breast, they use an infusion of the bark of the yuffo ; this is given

only every second morning, and proves gently emetic.

The following medicines, which are the chief remedies they employ in pectoral complaints, act either as emetics, or by exciting a slight degree of nausea. 1. Fundóoba, Timmanee: an infusion of the bark is drank every morning, and is much commended as an expectorant; in taste, it very much resembles juniper.

2. Mabamp, Timmanee, tamarind tree : an infusion of the leaves in boiling water is drank when cold, every morning, to promote expectoration in cases of shortness of breath; it tastes slightly acid, with a degree of astringency.

3. Bissay or Bissaing, Timmanee: an infusion of a handful of the leaves of this plant in boiling water, taken in the quantity of a tea-cupfull, produces full vomiting three or four times, after which it proves smartly purgative. It is a very strong and durable bitter, without possessing astringency. Sometimes they add to this plant an handful of the leaves of one called bakkarawóotoo, to increase its emetic powers.

The milky juice of gang-gáng taken in the quantity of half a table-spoonfull, proves gently emetic and purgative; when it has sufficiently operated, the juice of a lime immediately puts a stop to its action.

The bark of malip, or plum tree, is boiled in water, and frequently exhibited as an emetic; this effect is rendered more certain by the addition of a little of the bark of the kola and yuffo trees.

A decoction of the bark of a tree, called by the Timmanees moot, and by the Bulloms 'n-chok, is frequently used as an emetic, or, as they term it, to clean the stomach. The fruit of the same tree, when very young, is eaten in the morning, to remove nausea and sickness. From the seeds of this tree the natives obtain a kind of butter, as has been already mentioned.

A decoction of the leaves of the lime bush, called by the Timmanees limree, is frequently drank warm, in the morning, in the quantity of a tea-cupfull, when it proves emetic, and frequently purgative. This fragrant tree is greatly esteemed by the natives, and enters into the composition of several of their medicines. It was equally cele-brated among the ancients. Virgil thus describes its virtues :

> —————quo non præsentius ullum,
> Pocula siquando sævæ infecere novercæ,
> Miscueruntque herbas, & non innoxia verba,
> Auxilium venit, ac membris agit atra venena.
> —————*Folia haud ullis labentia ventis ;*
> Flos ad prima tenax : animas & olentia Medi
> Ora fovent illo, & senibus medicantur anhelis *.

Pliny likewise speaks of it in terms of praise, " Malus Assyria, quam alii vocant medicam, ve-nenis medetur. Odore præcellit foliorum quoque, qui transit in vestes una conditus arcetque ani-malium noxia †."

* Georg. ii. 127.   † Lib. xii. c. 7.

In cases of loss of appetite, they use a decoc
tion of the leaves of dakóona, so called by the
Soosoos and Timmanees, and by the Bulloms
lakóona: it is a very powerful bitter, somewhat
resembling wormwood, and is drank every morning. It is frequently mixed with honey, and
taken as an aphrodisiac.

When, together with a loss of appetite, there
is a bitter taste in the mouth, accompanied with
other symptoms of bile, a decoction of the leaves
of bullanta is recommended to be drank every
morning.

When the stomach is affected with indigestion,
and oppressed with a sense of weight, they make
use of a decoction of the roots of the following
plants : 1. Morronday. 2. Bangbee. 3. Demba-
eeree. 4. Dundakky. 5. The young palm-tree:
the roots are cut small, and a few unripe limes are
added, together with a little honey or sugar : this
medicine is given by cup-fulls, and proves briskly
purgative.

When any thing taken disagrees with the stomach, or when a poison has been swallowed
by design or accident, they use a very powerful
purgative, called by the Soosoos, tolinghee : the
outer skin of the root, which is a powerful astringent, is carefully scraped off, and thrown away;
the inner part is cut into small pieces, and
boiled with rice, or made into broth, with a
fowl, which is drank until the desired effect be
produced.

Upon the island of Bananas they have a very

violent purgative, which they call pulga-pootoo, or white man's physic, pootoo signifying a white man ; it is the same with the physic nut, jatropha cureas, in the West Indies, from whence it has probably been brought by Europeans. The purgative quality of the nut resides entirely in the corculum of the seed, and when this is removed, the cotyledons may be eaten with impunity, in any quantity : they resemble a sweet almond in taste. Five *whole* kernels are a sufficient dose for a strong man; in irritable and weak stomachs, when taken in greater quantity, they not only prove violently purgative, but produce severe vomiting, attended with a burning heat of the fauces. Ligon says, " I myselfe took five of them, and they gave me twelve vomits, and above twenty stooles *." The tree is chiefly used on the Bananas to make fences—According to Dr. Wright, a decoction of the *leaves* is often used with advantage in violent belly-achs, attended with vomiting. It is easier on the stomach than any thing else, and seldom fails to effect a discharge by stool. Lond. Med. Journal, vol. viii.

A captain of a vessel informed me, that having been seized with a spitting of blood, attended with a tickling cough, slight fever, and much restlessness and anxiety, he went on shore, among the natives on the Leeward Coast. The headman of the village was at the same time his host

---

* Hist. of Barbadoes.

and physician ; he spread for him upon the floor of
a hut, several beds, telling him that when tired
of one he must remove to another, until he felt
a disposition to sleep. An infusion of a plant
was occasionally administered, which excited gentle vomiting, and his diet consisted of fish, and
strong soups joined with mucilaginous herbs, by
which means in less than three weeks he was perfectly restored to health.

CHAP. VII.

GENERAL DISEASES.

DISEASES OF THE EYES. NYCTALOPIA. CASE OF
CROUP. SORE THROAT. CORPULENCY. SMALL-
POX. INOCULATION. MEASLES.

DISEASES of the EYES very rarely occur
upon the coast of Africa, notwithstanding
what has been alledged respecting the pernicious
effects of rice, their favourite food. Bontius says,
those who sail to Amboyna, Banda, and the Mo-
luccas, are frequently affected with weakness of
sight, and even total blindness, which is removed by a change of air, or a better diet. The
inhabitants of these islands, he adds, attribute
this complaint to the eating of hot rice; hence the
Javanese and Malays always expose the rice,
when just boiled, to a current of air. These noxious qualities of rice are attributed by Bontius
to its growing in wet and swampy places,
whereby it incorporates some marshy or fæcu-
lent substance, more penetrating in hot than in
cold rice; though, he says, the odour of even dry
and raw rice oppresses the head, and induces a degree of somnolency. It may be perhaps alleged
that, as the rice grows in the neighbourhood of Sierra
Leone in dry ground, and even upon the sides of

steep hills, it does not acquire these noxious qualities, of which the natives have not the smallest
dread. Whether under weakness of the eyes,
Bontius includes also the disease of nyctalopia,
or night blindness, which not unfrequently occurs
in warm climates, is uncertain. Of this latter
complaint, three or four instances came under
my observation, not among the natives, who do
not appear to know the disease, but among the
children of the Nova Scotia settlers in Free Town.
Two of these instances occurred in the same family, all the individuals of which were remarkable
for a peculiar prominence of the globe of the eye,
and a dilated pupil; in the other cases, no peculiarity was observable, nor could the disease be
attributed to any certain cause. It was of no long
continuance, and appeared to be carried off by
the exhibition of emetics and calomel purges.

Pliny takes notice of this disease, and recommends goat's liver to be eaten as a cure. Speaking
of these animals he says, tradunt & noctu non minus cernere, quam interdiu : ideo si caprinum
jecur vescantur, restitui verspertinam aciem his,
quos nyctalopas vocant. Lib. viii. c. 50.

The inhabitants of Syene in Egypt are, according to Mr. Bruce, affected with a weakness and
soreness of the eyes, terminating in blindness;
this is thought to be occasioned by the hot wind
of the desert.

The natives of Issinee, on the Gold Coast,
where rice is very little used for food, are liable
to inflammations of the eyes, which is attributed

to the great heat and glaring light of the rays of the sun reflected from the sandy soil *.

I have never seen an instance of blindness among the native Africans, except in very old people, who are not often affected with it; nor has an instance of obstinate opthalmia ever occurred to my notice. Their principal remedy for opthalmia, when it does occur, is pan-a-pánnee (Timmanee), tontáy, (Soosoo). The fruit, which is the part made use of, is shaped like a pear, but having a longer neck. When used, the apex is cut off, and a drop of the juice is pressed from it into the eye: I once saw it applied; it seemed to produce sharp pain, which continued only a few minutes. It is much commended in dimness of the cornea, and is also employed to remove specks or films. The juice is of an acid, and very astringent taste.

When the inflammation of the eye is very severe, it is usual to drop into it some milk from a woman's breast.

Another very celebrated remedy in opthalmia is a species of reed called by the Timmanees cattop; oo-sháa, (Bullom); kaymanghee (Soosoo). The stem is roasted over the fire, and a few drops of the juice, when milk warm, are squeezed into the eye. It produces a very acute pain for a short time. I saw it of use in scrophulous inflammation of the eye, opthalm. membran. The juice

* Isert. Reise nach Guinee.

is of an acid sweetish taste, and the stem is often chewed by the natives to quench their thirst. The leaves of this plant, first bruised in a mortar, and then heated over the fire, are applied hot to contused parts.

In slight cases of opthalmia the eye is washed with a decoction of the leaves of mekkamaken-zee.

A warm decoction of the leaves of a plant, called by the Timmanees yabákyaba, is used to wash the *stye* on the eyelids, hordeolum.

I have reason to suspect that an instance of the CROUP occurred at Free Town, in a stout boy about fifteen years old, a native of the Kroo coast ; but unfortunately the disease was neither suspected, nor was danger apprehended until the fatal termination took place, which was within forty-eight hours from his first complaining. There was a degree of tumefaction of the throat externally, reaching to the ears, and affecting a portion of the parotid gland on each side: he complained of an acute pain in the throat, rendering deglutition difficult ; but there was not any appearance of inflammation in the internal fauces. His voice was little affected, but his respiration became very difficult before he died. His pulse was small, but not much accelerated, nor was there any preternatural heat of the skin. The restlessness attending this complaint was so great, joined to an impatience of confinement, that he could not be prevailed upon to continue in bed, but walked about until within a few minutes of his death, which in a great measure took off the attention of those about him. Upon examining the seat of the disease after death, which was readily allowed by his countrymen, who seemed pleased that any attention was paid to the deceased, there was nothing more to be seen than a slight degree of redness in the upper part of the larynx, immediately below the epiglottis.

In SORE-THROAT, generally of the inflammatory kind, when attended with much tumefaction of the tonsils, and difficulty of swallowing, they use the young leaves of a small tree, called by the Soosoos wubbay, by the Timmanees apél, by the Bulloms pil, and by the Kroos ghéang : these are beaten up with some grains of malaguetta pepper, mixed with a little water, and given as a drink. This tree bears bunches of berries, resembling those of the common elder, at first red, but afterwards turning black. They contain a single seed, which is almost as hot as pepper. When the bark is cut, there exudes a gummi-resinous juice as red as blood.

In so hot a climate, it may appear strange for POLYSARCIA or CORPULENCY to occur as a disease. Among the Bulloms and Timmanees, the young people, especially the females, are rather full-formed and plump, than corpulent, but old persons are in general thin. Among the Mandingos corpulency is more frequent, and they endeavour

to obviate it by an infusion of the bark of a
tree, called by the Bulloms bal, by the Soosoos
shookay, and by the Timmanees obiss; it is bitter, but has no sensible effect. This tree produces a rough brown plum, which has a sweet
taste, and is often used to make a kind of beer.
The unripe fruit has a narcotic quality, and
induces considerable nausea. Brisk purgatives
are occasionally employed with a view to diminish
corpulency. Profuse sweating is also made use
of for this purpose, and the patient sits over a decoction of ginsee-ginse, while the steam is confined
by a thick cotton cloth thrown over him. The
same infusion is used, when cold, as a wash for
the body during the day.

The SMALL POX, from the concurrent testimony
of authors, is a further addition to the diseases
supposed to have originated in Africa, terra
ferace veneni. Whether it first began in Ethiopia or Arabia is uncertain; but from the latter country it was imported into Europe. Dr.
Friend supposed that this disease took its rise
in Egypt, because Rhazes informs us that a physician of the name of Aaron, who was born at
Alexandria, and practised in the reign of Mohammed, about the year 622, had treated of
this disease; but its origin is carried farther
back by Professor Reiske, who says he read
the following words in an old Arabic manu-
script, in the public library at Leyden. " This
year, in fine, 572, the birth of Mohammed, the

small pox and measles made their first appearance
in Arabia *." Dr. Mead adds, respecting the
small pox, " I really take this disease to be a
plague of its own kind, which was originally bred
in Africa, and more especially in Ethiopia, as the
heat is excessive there ; and thence, like the true
plague, was brought into Arabia and Egypt †."
However just these speculations may be, it is
certain, that at the present day, the small-pox is
so far from being endemial on the western coast
of Africa, on the windward part of it at least, that
it is always imported thither by Europeans. It is
called by the Timmanees oo-bumbo, by the Bulloms ka-bumbo, by the Soosoos kaka, and by the
Mandingos cassimasinghee. It is about twelve
years since its last appearance in the river Sierra
Leone, or on the Bullom shore. It was very fatal
in the higher branches of the river Sierra Leone,
in the year 1773, and about seventeen years
ago it appeared in the river Sherbro,' where it
proved very fatal, especially to old people.

It is upwards of twenty years since this disease
shewed itself in the Foola country : the Foolas
say it was at that time imported by an American vessel, which came to Rocundy, and add,
that many of the old people fell a sacrifice to
it. Among all the tribes near the coast there
is a great similarity in the mode of treating
the small pox. From the time of the eruption,

* Mead's Works.　　† Ibid.

which is generally towards the end of the third
day, the patient is not washed until the suppuration be completed ; for they suppose if cold
water were used to wash a person in this disease,
it would throw the matter upon the internal parts,
and prove fatal. As soon as matter appears in
the pustules, it is let out by a sharp pointed stick,
the pustule itself is removed, and after being well
washed with warm water, the sores are sprinkled
with the fine meal of the pigeon pea, called by
the Bulloms see-ti'l. This practice of removing
the pustule, however, is nòt general ; in some parts
of the country, they merely let out the matter,
and then wash the pustule well with warm water;
and as often as the pustule fills with matter, it is
opened and washed. Their hope of preventing the
face from being marked, rests upon their washing
and emptying the pustules very diligently. The
appearance of this disease excites a general alarm:
when any one is seized with it, he is immediately
removed to a place built for the purpose in the
woods, where no person is allowed to visit him,
but such as have had the disorder. A quantity
of fine sand is spread upon the ground, on which
are laid cloths to serve for the patient's bed. The
diet is restricted to milk, thin soups, and lean
meat ; nothing cold is allowed for drink. The
chief medicine made use of is an infusion of a
plant that tastes like sorrel, called by the Mandingos santoo, by the Foolas folleree, and by the
Soosoos da ; hibiscus, tea plant. When the pus-

tules are dry, and begin to desquamate, the patient is washed, and his body anointed with some soft ointment.

The practice of inoculation is totally unknown in the neighbourhood of Sierra Leone, where, if ever practised, it has been by Europeans alone. The small pox is said to do little mischief in Morocco, " because of the temperance of the climate, and the abstinence of the people." They are acquainted with inoculation in the *interior parts* of the country * ; but the Moors do not inoculate, " except those who live on the mountains, the Brebes and the Shellu of the south (or aborigines) — hence it may be concluded that the small-pox was known in Africa before the invasion of the Arabs, and that the mode of communicating it by insertion must have been more ancient in these countries than Mahometanism ; because, however powerful the ascendant of religion may be, it is very slow in rooting out the prejudices and customs of nations †." In the Medical Observations and Inquiries, vol. i. it is asserted, upon the testimony of some negroes in America, that inoculation is commonly practised in Africa, so that old people seldom have the disease ; it is added, " they generally inoculate all their young, as soon as the infection comes into the neighbourhood. —— In the regimen

* Mr. Park informs us that the negroes on the Gambia practise inoculation for the small-pox.

† Chemier's present State of Morocco.

under it, they only abstain from all flesh meat, and
drink plentifully of water acidulated with the juice
of limes, which grow large and plentifully in their
country." Inoculation has been frequently practised to a considerable extent on board of slave
vessels, and though no instance has fallen under
my observation, it has always proved successful.
An ingenious writer observes, that " the small
pox in cold countries is more fatal to blacks * than
to whites. In the Boston small pox, of 1752,
there died whites in the natural way about one in
eleven, but one in eighty by inoculation ; blacks in
the natural way, one in eight ; by inoculation one
in twenty. In hot countries it is more fatal to
whites than blacks. In Charles Town, South Ca-
rolina, when the small pox prevailed, 1738, it was
found, upon a scrutiny, that in the natural way,
of 647 whites died 157, one in four ; by inoculation of 156 whites, died nine, or one in twenty ;
of 1024 blacks in the natural way there died 138,
one in seven and half ; of 251 blacks, by inoculation there died seven, one in thirty-six †." The
same author, speaking of the manner in which the
North American Indians treat this disease, says,
" their principal remedy is sweating in huts warmed by heated stones, and thereupon immediate
immersion in cold water. In inflammatory and
eruptive epidemical fevers, e. g. small pox, this
practice depopulates them "

* An affecting instance of this is related in Cartwright's History of Labradore.
† Douglas's Polit. Survey, ii. 398.

Notwithstanding THE MEASLES are said to be of African origin, I could not obtain from the natives any satisfactory account of the disease, because it is difficult to make them comprehend by words alone the object of your enquiry. I was informed by a native in the Rio Pongas, of Portuguese extraction, who spoke remarkably good English, that they have sometimes an eruptive disease appearing among them as an epidemic, which he called fundoo, in Soosoo foondaing. He said, it is preceded by a sensation of cold, followed by heat, and attended with a cough and watery eyes; it is not dangerous, and runs its course in a few days. For the cure, they rub the body all over with the fine flour of rice, which is sometimes mixed with honey. This person's character for dishonesty induced me to pay little credit to his account; but I have been assured by a captain of a vessel, a man of probity and good information, who had been frequently on the coast, that the measles were once brought on board a slave ship in which he was, by a canoe from Cape Coast, and that one of the men in the canoe was ill of the complaint. The infection spread immediately, and several slaves were taken ill, but by separating them from those in health, the disease was speedily checked. It proved to be very mild, and had probably been imported by some vessel trading on the coast.

The old Portuguese abovementioned, took notice of a disease which he said he had seen, though rarely, and which appears to resemble pemphigus.

He called it fook-salabrass. By the Soosoos and Mandingos, he said, it is called bombórrassoo, and by the Bulloms baárra. This disease is preceded by slight cold, followed by heat, after which large vesicles appear, resembling those occasioned by a burn or scald. They puncture the vesicle, and when the water is discharged they wash the sore with a decoction of the bark of tolinghee or yecre scraped fine.

CHAP. VIII.

GENERAL DISEASES.

YAWS

OF all the diseases which are supposed to have originated in Africa, the only one which can be said with any degree of certainty to be indigenous in that continent is the YAWS. It frequently occurs among the slaves in the West India islands and America, by whom it has been imported from Africa into those countries; it is almost unknown in Europe, for though it has sometimes been imported, it has never spread.

The yaws is called by the Bulloms bihl, by the Timmanees tirree or catirree, by the Mandingos mansera, and by the Soosoos dokkettee or kota. It is called by the Portuguese on the coast boba, and by the French pianes.

This complaint is usually preceded by violent pains of the limbs, which somewhat resemble those of rheumatism, and are particularly severe round the joints; these pains are attended with much languor and debility, and frequently continue several days without any further appearance of disease. These precursory symptoms are succeeded by a degree of pyrexia, sometimes attended with rigor, though in other instances the fever is slight and scarcely noticed.

For the most part the patient complains of head-ach, loss of appetite, and pains of the back and loins, which are exacerbated towards evening. When these symptoms have continued a few days, they are followed by an eruption of pustules, more or less numerous, which appear in various parts of the body, but especially upon the forehead, face, neck, groin, pudenda, and round the anus. The eruption of these pustules is not completed over the whole body at one time, neither do they shew themselves in any regular succession on the different parts; but while one crop is falling off, another is making its appearance in another place Every fresh eruption of pustules is preceded by a slight febrile paroxysm. The pustules are filled with an opake whitish fluid; they are, at their first appearance, not so large as the head of a small pin, but gradually grow larger, until they attain the size of a sixpence, or even of a shilling. When the pustules burst, a thick viscid matter is discharged, which forms a foul and dense crust or scab upon the surface. In general, the number and size of the pustules is proportioned to the degree of eruptive fever; when the febrile symptoms are slight, there are few pustules, but they are mostly of a larger size than when the complaint is more violent and extensive. From the larger kind of pustules there frequently arise red fungous excrescences of various magnitudes, from the size of a pea

to that of a large mulberry, which fruit, owing to
their rough, granulated surfaces, they somewhat
resemble. These fungi, though they rise considerably above the surface of the skin, have but a small
degree of sensibility ; they never suppurate kindly,
but gradually discharge a sordid glutinous fluid,
which forms an ugly scab round the edges of the
excrescence, and covers the upper part of it, when
much elevated, with white sloughs. When these
eruptions appear upon any part of the body covered with hair, the colour of the hair is gradually
changed from black to white.

It sometimes happens at the commencement
of the disease, when the pustules are few, that
there is some doubt respecting the nature of the
complaint: to determine this, the natives open one
of the pustules, and drop upon it a little of the
juice of the capsicum ; if it be of the yaw species
little or no pain is excited.

This disease is communicable in every way in
which syphilis can be produced, though it is less
frequently contracted by coition ; because, as the
complaint can only affect the same person *once*
in his lifetime, and as in Africa it is usually gone
through in childhood, of course this mode of pro-
pagating it is in a great measure prevented.
The disease never spreads by miasmata floating
in the air : it can only be communicated by the
application of matter from a yaw pustule or sore
to a wound in a person who has not previously
laboured under the disease. The complaint is
sometimes inoculated by means of a large fly,

called in the West Indies the yaw fly. When this insect alights upon a running yaw, which the Africans never keep covered, and afterwards settles upon the body of an uninfected person, it introduces the poison, if there happen to be a wound or scratch there, as effectually as the most dexterous surgeon.

Dr. Bancroft says, " none ever receive this disorder, whose skins are whole ; for which reason the whites are rarely infected ; but the backs of the negroes being often raw by whipping, and suffered to remain naked, they scarce ever escape it *."

Doctor Mosely, in his elaborate treatise on sugar, asserts, that " there are several distempers of bestial origin," and is of opinion the " yaws is one of them." It is to be regretted that Dr. Mosely has not treated more fully on this disease, as few persons have had greater opportunities of observation, or of turning them to profit. Whether, from what is said above, Dr. Mosely imagines the yaws to have originated in consequence of a " bestial humour" being introduced into the human body, like the matter of the cow pox, or whether he supposes that the disease arose ex concubitu virorum cum simiis, as some old authors have strangely imagined, is not very evident. The doctor has certainly committed a slight error when he says, that the yaws " breaks out in negroes without any

* Hist. of Guiana.

communication, society, or contact," and that
" the seeds of the yaws descend from those
who have ever had it to their latest posterity."
This is so far from being the case in Africa,
and it is to be hoped in the West Indies also,
that in no instance whatever does the disease
arise except from the application of the contagious matter of yaws to a person who has not
previously been affected with it. Neither is there
more reason to suppose that the seeds of this
disorder are transmitted to posterity by hereditary descent, than that the contagion of the small
pox, measles, or any other of the exanthemata,
are communicated hereditarily.

The pustules generally appear first upon that
part of the body where the contagious matter
has been introduced, though I cannot, from my
own observation, determine, since the disease
so rarely happens in Africa to adults, whether
primary ulcers shew themselves on the pudenda,
when the disease has been contracted by venereal connection : it is very usual, however, after
the system has been infected, for ulcers to appear
on those parts, as is frequently seen in children.
Buboes rarely or never occur. When there is
an ulcer or a slight wound in any part, the pustules either appear there first, or are more copious there than elsewhere ; the surface of the sore
or ulcer also changes from an healthy appearance
to a foul and sloughy state, the granulations become pale and spongy, and the purulent discharge
is changed to ichor.

The duration of the complaint is very uncertain, but it depends in some degree upon the complete eruption of the pustules : this, as has been said, is not completed at once, but may take up several weeks or months ; when no more pustules are thrown out, and when those already upon the skin no longer increase in size, the disease is supposed to have reached its acme. About this time it happens, on some part of the body or other, that one of the pustules becomes much larger than the rest, equalling or surpassing the size of an half crown piece : it assumes the appearance of an ulcer, and instead of being elevated above the skin like others, it is considerably depressed ; the surface is foul and sloughy, and pours out an ill conditioned ichor, which spreads very much, by corroding the surrounding sound skin : this is what is called the *master* or *mother yaw*. If proper attention be not paid to keep the surface of the ulcer clean by daily washing, the matter becomes very acrid, and when near a bone sometimes affects it with caries.

When the fungous or mulberry-like excrescences appear upon the soles of the feet, they are prevented from rising by the resistance of the thick hard epidermis, and give so much pain that the person affected is unable to walk. The fungi thus situated are called by the negroes in the West Indies *tubba*, or crab yaws. They are sometimes so large as to cover a great part of the sole of the foot ; at other times, they are not larger than a shilling : they are frequently affected, like corns, by different states of the atmosphere, especially by rainy weather.

The yaw pustules are in general largest upon the face, in the axillæ, groins, perinæum, and round the anus. The itch or cracraws, as it is called in Africa, is sometimes mistaken for the yaws; but in the latter complaint, the ulcers are more elevated than those of the itch; they also appear in the face, and are generally devoid of itchiness.

The learned M. Sauvages has unnecessarily distinguished this disease into two species, the framboesia guineensis and framboesia americana, the disease being precisely the same whether it appear in Africa, or the West Indies, &c.

Professor Sprengel has, on no better grounds, made a similar division of this disease into " yaws and pians:" the former, he says, has been described by the Arabians under the title safath. In the middle ages, it was sometimes called variola magna, as it seemed to differ from small pox only in being a chronic disease. The pians, he says, has been improperly included with the former under the term framboesia, although it has not been so extensively diffused as the yaws. Prof. Sprengel adds, that it was originally endemic in one district of the coast of Guinea, the kingdom of Sanguin, and that it is not so readily communicated to the whites as the yaws[*].

* Rurt Sprengels Handbüch der Pathologie

It has been asserted by some authors, that Europeans are not liable to this complaint, but I have known several instances of it among them. The following case happened in the person of an European, a slave trader in the Rio Nunez. In the month of July, 1793, whilst in perfect health, he was suddenly seized with severe pains in the joints of his whole body, particularly in those of his arms and knees. The pains were greatly aggravated by external heat, especially at night by the warmth of bed: they were also exasperated by rubbing the affected parts with oil, and other emollient applications. The only relief he could obtain was by plunging his body into cold water, which procured an immediate, though only a temporary remission of pain; so that he was obliged to repeat it four or five times during the night. At the end of a week or ten days, the pains became less severe, and recurred less frequently. About this time pustules, which remained always distinct, broke out over his whole body; they were not very numerous, but were most troublesome as well as most plentiful upon his legs. He then applied to an old woman celebrated for her skill in this disease, and during two months which he continued under her care, he swallowed a great quantity of decoctions of herbs, without experiencing the least relief. Being tired with this ill success, he began to use mercury, first in small doses, as an alterative, and afterwards on a different plan, so as to excite a gentle salivation. This course had no apparent effect upon the disease, but he felt greatly debilitated in consequence of it. During the process, the pustules continued to dry and fall off in one place, and to break out in another: six weeks or two months usually elapsed between the first appearance of the pustules and their falling off. There were no depressions or discolourations observable in the skin on any part of the body after the desquamation of the pustules, except upon the legs, and in them alone was any degree of pain or trouble excited. When a spot broke out upon the legs, it degenerated into a troublesome ulcer, which could only be brought to heal by the application of strong escharotics. During all the time of his being affected with this disorder, his joints felt remarkably stiff, with a sensation as if some foreign body were contained within the articulation ; or, as if the joints did not move with freedom, through a deficiency of synovia: this was especially felt in the knees. At the time he gave this account, Sept. 23, 1795, the stiffness was so great, that after sitting awhile, he had scarcely sufficient strength to raise himself up and bend his knees. His skin likewise acquired a remarkable and disagreeable increase of sensibility, and he still complains of a painful tenderness of the integuments over his whole body, insomuch that a gentle tap produces as violent a sensation as a smart blow would have excited formerly. This has been the case ever since he became affected with the disease. He experiences an increased quickness of pulse towards evening, and not unfrequently has a degree of fever and restlessness during the early part of the night. These febrile symptoms appear to depend upon the degree of debility induced in consequence of the disease. His legs are much swoln, and are greatly discoloured, being of a dark brown colour. This change of colour occurred during the present disease, after an attack of common remittent fever, attended with profuse night sweats. One evening he complained of an unusual degree of heat and pain in his legs, which he found, on uncovering them, to be changed, from the calf of the leg to the toes, to nearly the colour of a black man's skin. He still has a small ulcer upon his leg, which, he thinks, is a remnant of the yaws. During the course of the disease he had a severe sore throat, but this he did not attribute to the yaws, nor does he think that hoarseness is an attendant symptom. He is of opinion that the natives have no cure for yaws, but that it is effected always by nature *.

I saw a man labouring under this disease, toge-

* The yaws is not mentioned by authors as a disease which occurs in Egypt, though from the frequent communication of that country with those parts of Africa in which the disease is endemial, we might be led to suspect it would be imported. There is reason, however, to suppose that the yaws does actually appear there, though mistaken for the venereal disease; this will appear evident from the following case, extracted from a recent publication, where it is given as an instance of syphilis. "The natives, (of Egypt) who are unacquainted with the use of mercury,

ther with two of his children, who appeared to be between six and eight years of age. The children had been affected about eight months, but the man only four or five. In the latter, pain of the head, sickness at stomach, and general uneasiness, had preceded the eruption for a day or two. The pustules first appeared upon the outside of one of his thighs; they were very numerous, and of a small kind, never throwing out fungi. He experienced severe pains in his joints, which were much aggravated by heat, and relieved by cold. In many parts the pustules were quite dry, and,

and indeed of minerals in general, as employed internally, are yet provided, as they say, with efficacious remedies for the venereal disease. They use flax oil, fresh, as it is expressed from the seed. A Greek, who was in the service of Murad Bey as a mariner, *(Galeongi)*, and who was known to me in Kahira, had been infected, and on applying to a Frank physician, was told that it would be necessary immediately to use mercurials. The man was not inclined to confinement or to regimen, and went to a Copt at Jizé, who professed to relieve the sick. This man ordered him to take two coffee-cups of flax oil every morning fasting, and directed no regimen, but that of keeping himself warm. The Greek observed none, for he continued freely the use of *aqua vitæ*, and even sacrificed to Venus, (for persons who have been once infected, and fully cured, are, it is said, in no fear of re-infection), and was often in the heat of the sun. He had continued this method for two months, when a general eruption took place over his body, but chiefly about the head and glands of the throat. In this condition I saw him. His Æsculapius ordered him to cover the pustules of his face with a kind of red earth, found in some parts of Egypt. They gradually became dry, and came off without leaving any mark. At the end of the third month from the time he had applied to the Copt, and one month after the appearance of the eruption, the man was in perfect health, and the skin had completely recovered its tone and polish." Browne's Travels in Africa, Egypt, and Syria.

where scratched, fell off, leaving the skin quite clear beneath. A kind of fungous excrescence had appeared some time before within one of his nostrils, and had given him much pain, especially at nights, but was gone when I saw him. The alæ nasi and cheeks had been covered with the same kind of eruption as that on his body, but the dried pustules had fallen off. He complained at this time of nothing, but of extreme debility, though apparently robust and in good health; the pains in his joints, even in those of his fingers, were also severe.

The back and sides of one of the children were covered with irregular clusters of pustules, very much resembling those in the shingles, except that the pustules were not so pellucid, nor was the skin inflamed. In this child, as well as in the father, the pustules did not grow large and throw out fungous excrescences, but after continuing stationary for some time, they dried and fell off; they were very numerous on her face and neck. In the other child, who had been ill about a month longer than the last, the pustules were of a large kind, and were covered with a foul yellow crust.

In the following instance both kinds of pustules occurred: the person appeared to be about thirty years of age, and had been affected nine months with this complaint. There were about forty or fifty pustules upon his face, nearly resembling, as to size and appearance, the pustules in the distinct small pox when fully maturated, but with no inflammation round their base. His arms and body were likewise covered with the same kind of pustules. In some parts of the back there appeared several small, flat, semi-pellucid pustules, surrounded and intermixed with those of the usual size. In the axillæ there were six or eight irregular crusts or eschars about the size of a shilling, from which the mulberry excrescences had sprung up, but they were now turned black by the application of lime juice and iron, which had been used to destroy them.

The pustules have not any fixed period, within which they dry and fall off. They leave no depression of the skin, but occasion a deeper tinge of black, which disappears in time. Several of the dried pustules had fallen off his face, none of which had reached a larger size than that of a common pea. Many large crusts appeared upon his body, but they were nearly dried up by the astringent applications made use of; there were none upon his legs, but the vestiges of them were marked by an increased blackness in various places. The crusts or eschars dried up always at the centre, and in a very irregular manner: some of them had this appearance :

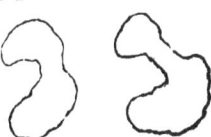

Upon his thighs some crusts still remained. The disease first made its appearance in a pustule upon the little toe of the left foot, which has long been well; from the foot it affected the legs, then the back of the neck, head, face, arms, and body. Almost all the first crop of pustules have fallen off, and have been succeeded by a fresh eruption; but he remarked that a new pustule never appeared upon the same spot which had already thrown out one. He complained of great weakness and pains in his joints, particularly in those of his arms, shoulders, and knees. The pains were greatly aggravated at nights. In other respects he appeared to enjoy perfect health, and had no sickness previously to the eruption.

This disease has not received that attention from medical practitioners which its importance demands; for on account of its disgusting appearance, and the danger arising from too close a survey, the treatment of it has been chiefly trusted to ignorant people. Hence the description of yaws has been very imperfect, and still remains unsatisfactory. Nosologists have, in consequence of this defective history of the disease, been induced to class it with scrophula, syphilis, elephantiasis, &c. diseases to which it bears a very slight and distant analogy. On the contrary, if its stages of eruption, maturation, and desquamation be considered, though not strictly agreeing as to time with other eruptive diseases; and if to this be added that it never affects the same individual twice, we cannot hesitate to place it among the exanthemata.

The yaws has likewise been confounded with other complaints. Sydenham supposes the yaws to be the same disease as the lues venerea, and that it was brought into Europe by the Spaniards, who were infected by the negroes purchased in Africa; " apud quos invaluit mos ille barbarus homines Europæis mercibus permutandi *."

Dr. Hillary † is of opinion that it has been described by Hali Abbas al Magiouschi, or the Magus, as he was surnamed from his learning, under the title lepra, and in the following words:

* Epistola ad Henr. Paman, M. D.

The writer of the article Epian, in the Encyclopedie Methodique, has likewise classed the yaws and venereal disease as similar complaints. " Epian. Nom que les naturels de Sainte Domingue donnoient à la verole, qu'on croit avoir été endemique dans cette isle, & qui parut pour la premier fois en Europe l'an 1494. Quelques-uns ont cru que c'étoit un caractère de maladie plus grave & plus facheux encore que la verole ; mais il est actuellement prouvé, que c'est la meme maladie que les François ont appellè Mal de Naples, et les Italiens Mal François, chacun s'empressant de desavouer l'origine d'un mal aussi honteux, et accusant ses voisins d'en avoir propagé la contagion." Tom. vi. p. 2.

There is, however, one circumstance, which, if founded on fact, will sufficiently discriminate the yaws from every modification of syphilis, and from the whole class of exanthemata. It is asserted by Bajon [1], that the virus of yaws is capable of being communicated to domestic animals ; and when it appears among the fowls, the disease spreads so rapidly, that to check it, those affected with the complaint must be immediately killed. Dogs are equally liable to be affected, and in these animals it assumes very much the appearance of the venereal disease. We know from experiments instituted for the purpose, that the constitution of brutes is unsusceptible of the variolous, morbillous, syphilitic, and some other contagions to which the human subject is liable.

† Halleri Bib. Med. Pract.

[1] Geschichte von Cayenne.

" Lepra albedo est quæ in exterioribus fit cutis: et aliquando in quibusdam sine aliis est membris: nonnunquam vero in toto fit corpore, interdum ut fit corporis color albus. Quæ in membro est, si ex mala fit frigida complexione, hæc sunt signa; quum membrum in quo est, album est colore, itidemque ejus pili; & si cutis phlebotomo vel certe acie pungitur, sanguis ab eo non egreditur, sed humiditas alba *." In this very brief account there is nothing characteristic of this disease, which exhibits peculiarities sufficiently striking to have excited the attention of less accurate observers. Dr. Hillary, and some others, are also of opinion, that the yaws is the leprosy described by Moses; but it is enough to read the description of the two complaints to be convinced of their difference.

There is a modification of the venereal disease met with in Scotland which is called sivvens, or sibbens, from a word in the Scoto-Saxon language, spoken in the Highlands, signifying a wild raspberry; in Gaelic or Erse it is called soucruu †. In some parts it is also called the *yaws*, from a fancied resemblance to the disease of that name. The sibbens, however, does not, like the yaws, appear only once in the same person, but may occur as often as the venereal disease. These three complaints are all communicable by similar means; but the sibbens more frequently takes

---

* Theorice, cap. xvi. lib. 8.   † Hill's Cases in Surgery.

place after eating or drinking out of the vessel used by an infected person, in which case small ulcerations appear within the mouth and fauces, having precisely the character of venereal ulcers, and very speedily affecting the bones of the palate and nose, afterwards those of the face, and of other parts of the body.

There are but two appearances in which sibbens and yaws can be said to bear any resemblance to each other. When the former disease is received into the system otherwise than by the mouth, it appears as a cutaneous complaint, breaking out in a number of small itchy pustules. But the chief characteristic of the sibbens, and that in which it most resembles the yaws, is an eruption of soft spongy excrescences, like raspberries, which appear in various parts of the body, especially round the anus : they rise considerably above the surface of the skin, but are more painful than the yaw-pustules. They do not, like the yaws, admit of a natural cure, but continue to spread indefinitely. Escharotics are insufficient to remove them, but they speedily disappear by the exhibition of mercury. The itch, yaws, and sibbens, have this in common, that they most readily affect the lower classes, or those who pay little attention to cleanliness. The venereal disease and yaws are frequently seen at one time in the same person, and according to Schilling *, we have an

* Godfr. Wilh. Schilling de Morbo in Europa pene ignoto, quem Americani vocant yaws.

instance of even *three specific diseases* occurring at the same time, lepra, framboesia, and small pox.

The yaws is said to be rendered more mild in its symptoms, and quicker in its progress, by means of inoculation, a practice totally unknown to the natives round Sierra Leone. Mr. Edwards * was informed by a black woman wno came from Annamaboo, " that the natives on the Gold Coast give their children the *yaws*, (a frightful disorder) *by inoculation* ; and she described the manner of performing the operation to be making an incision in the thigh, and putting in some of the infectious matter. I asked her what benefit they expected from this practice ? She answered, that by this means their infants had the disorder slightly, and recovered speedily ; whereas by catching it at a later time of life, the disease, she said, ' got into the bone,' that was her expression."

The natives never attempt to cure this disease until it has nearly reached its height, when the fungi have acquired their full size, and no more pustules appear. One of their remedies is the bark of a tree, called by the Bulloms yuffo : this is boiled in water, and made stronger or weaker, according to the age of the patient. Some of this decoction is mixed with rice, and given for two succeeding mornings : it is then omitted for a week, and again exhibited two mornings to-

* History of the West Indies.

gether. It proves gently purgative. The ulcers are likewise washed every second day with a strong decoction of the same bark; and when this is done, the crusts are carefully removed from the surface of the sore. An infusion of the bark of bullanta is also used to wash the ulcers in yaws. The juice which exudes from the stem of nintee, when cut, is taken internally every morning in the quantity of a glassful; it possesses a degree of astringency, but produces no sensible effects. A decoction of the leaves of this plant is likewise used to wash the ulcers.

It has been already said, that one or more of the yaws usually acquires a larger size than the rest, and is called mother yaw, to destroy which recourse is had to more powerful means. Their most frequent application is lime-juice and iron: for this purpose an iron bar is heated red hot, and rubbed with a lime cut in two, the *boiling* juice of which falls immediately upon the sore; this, as may be imagined, produces excessive pain. Sometimes the rust of iron is boiled in lime juice, to which is added a quantity of the common black ants, or a certain proportion of Malaguetta pepper; and as in the former instance, the liquor is applied hot to the sore. It acts as an escharotic, and produces a crust upon the surface of the sore which is removed every second day.

In general, those who are of a lax and delicate habit of body are observed to have the yaws more favourably than the robust; hence women and children, provided they be in good health, suffer least from the disease. In children the duration of the yaws is from six to nine months, and in in Africa the disease is thought not less peculiar to childhood than the small pox is in Europe, but with this advantage, that they do not dread any fatal consequences from it. In adults the disease is seldom cured in less than a year, and sometimes takes up two or three; it affects them also more severely than children, and when they are somewhat advanced in age, often proves fatal.

It is usual in the West Indies to give medicines with a view of producing determination to the skin, and of assisting the expulsion of the morbific matter of the yaws. Agreeably to this theory, the remedies employed are either mercurials or antimonials in small doses; of the former, corrosive sublimate and calomel have been chiefly employed, or the inert combinations of mercury with sulphur. Sulphur, camphor, and guaiacum have been applied with the same intention; also decoctions of sarsaparilla, and the tepid bath. Perhaps the best and only safe means of conducting the disease to its height is, by a nourishing diet, by exercise proportioned to the patient's strength, by comfortable dry lodgings, with such other means as tend to invigorate the system. When the disease appears at a stand, mercury is in general had recourse to, either taken internally, or applied by inunction to the skin. Dr. Bancroft recommends mercury and camphor combined, and used so as to excite no sensible evacuation, but along with some sudorific to determine its effects to the skin. Dr. Schilling, in his learned and valuable Treatise de Framboesia, recommends mercury only in the latter period of the disease, when there are deep seated pains of the bones aggravated at night. He tried the solution of corrosive sublimate, as recommended by Van Swieten, in four patients, who had been ill nine months, and who had very large pustules. The season was cold and rainy, which he always found to aggravate the disease, and even to occasion the death of many patients at Surinam. In the above patients the decoct. lignor. was joined with the subl. solution; and they were made to use the exercise of sawing until fatigued. The medicine excited vomiting. After continuing its use for eight days, three of them were salivated, when the mercury was omitted, and the decoction continued alone, by which means they were cured in *three weeks.* No pain, nor inconvenience were experienced during the salivation, nor afterwards. The fourth patient could not be made to salivate, although he took double the quantity of mercury; he was, however, cured of his complaint. Dr. Wright, of Jamaica, after informing us that the yaws produce the same dreadful effects on the limbs, nose, and throat as the venereal disease, adds, that they are curable by mercurial alteratives and diaphoretic decoctions. " Of all the preparations of mercury, he continues, the corrosive sublimate appears to me to be the best for curing such inveterate disorders, especially when accompanied with such medicines as promote its natural tendency to the skin. Of this sort is guaiacum and sarsaparilla. I have found the following formula the best:

> Gum guaiacum, ten drachms.
> Virginia snake root, three drachms.
> Pimento, two drachms.
> Opium, one drachm.
> Corrosive sublimate, half a drachm.
> Proof spirits, two pounds.

To be mixed and digested for three days, and then strained.

Two tea-spoonfuls of this tincture given in half a pint of sarsaparilla decoction twice a day, will, in general, remove every symptom of lues or yaws in four or five weeks."

When mercury has been prematurely used, though it causes the pustules to fall off, and clears the skin, yet it does not cure the disease. A train of disagreeable symptoms sooner or later appear, which often continue to harass the patient during the miserable remnant of his life; this is called by the negroes the bone-ach. The unhappy sufferer is tormented with deep seated pains in the bones, especially round the joints, which are occasionally aggravated to a violent degree: the periosteum becomes thickened, inflamed, and painful, and nodes are formed on the bones. When these symptoms have continued for some time, the bones are affected with caries, and even become soft, and lose their form.

Escharotics are made use of to destroy the mother yaws, and of these the red precipitate is one of the best. A solution of corrosive sublimate and sal ammoniac in water is a very effectual lotion for the purpose; or they may be touched with a solution of a drachm of corrosive sublimate in an ounce of spirit of wine. The fungous excrescences on the soles of the feet, called crab yaws *, often prove very obstinate, and remain a long time after the disease has totally disappeared in other parts. They are only to be cured by the use of strong caustics. Dr. Moseley recommends for this purpose " to pare off the top of the yaw, and then lay upon it a diachylon with gum plaister sprinkled with the

---

* Dr. Chisholm mentions a very easy and effectual mode of extirpating those troublesome and obstinate fungi, the tubboes or crab yaws, by means of the juice of the manchineel apple in a state of vapour. For this purpose, " a hole large enough being dug in the sand, alternate layers of charcoal and manchineel apples are laid in it. When the charcoal is well lighted, and a thick smoke arises, the patient is made to place the diseased foot over it; and a piece of thick osnaburgh is laid over all, to prevent the escape of the vapour. At the end of an hour the foot is removed, and the crabs, which before the application of the steam were hard and untractable, are now completely rotten, insomuch that without giving the least pain, they are picked out with a small pointed knife." It may not be improper to add here from the same author, that he has repeatedly seen the dangerous effects of the poisonous manchineel removed by sea water, to which the bignonia leucoxylon (the white cedar of the country) is said to be also a certain antidote."

corrosive sublimate powdered, the size of the yaw, and let it remain for two or three days.—— On taking off the plaister, the yaw generally comes out like a plug; if not, it digests out in a day or two, with common dressings, and the part soon gets well *." On the contrary, Dr. Schilling recommends that equal parts of red precipitate and white vitriol should be sprinkled upon the yaw ; he dissuades from the use of corrosive sublimate or arsenic, having seen violent symptoms produced by their application.

* Treatise on Tropical Diseases.

CHAP. IX.

GENERAL DISEASES.

HERPES is not unfrequently met with among the Africans, particularly the species called serpigo or ring worm. It changes the skin in black persons to a copper colour. This complaint is called by the Soosoos and Mandingos muntay, and by the Timmanees munta. In order to cure it, they scrape the diseased part with a piece of stick, until the blood flow pretty freely; and then wash it with a decoction of the bruised leaves of a plant called by the Soosoos bangbee, to which is added a little salt and lime juice. This practice is repeated every day until the cure be completed. The flowers of the French guava tree, when bruised, yield an astringent juice, which is considered as a specific in this complaint *.

Dr. Wright † informs us, that " tetters, or ring-worms, are frequent amongst the black people in Jamaica, and amongst the Spaniards in America very inveterate. I have seen this complaint so universal, that the habit was tainted; the skin looked leprous, and the unhappy patient

* Bancroft. Hillary.
† Essays on the Malignant Fever of the West Indies.

had not a moment's ease from the intolerable itching or painful ulcers."

In the beginning, a poultice of the flowers of the ring-worm bush, French guayava tree, cassia alata, is of service, as are also sulphureous applications; but, in more advanced stages of the disease, mercurials externally, and the decoction of woods taken inwardly, give the only chance of a cure *."

According to Piso † the leaves of the ricinus macerated in water or vinegar, are of great use in herpetic eruptions.

KRA-KRA is an Ebo word, corrupted, as I have been informed, from kra-thra, which signifies the itch. Although every nation on the coast distinguishes this disease by a peculiar name, yet the term kra-kra pervades the whole; it has been introduced probably by Europeans from the West Indies, where Ebo slaves are held in the highest estimation: hence it is likely their language should predominate, and give origin to many cant phrases in those islands.

This disorder is called by the Mandingos cattee, by the Soosoos cashee, by the Timmanees tobul, and by the Bulloms ee-shok-kil. As they do not look upon the kra-kras to be infectious, they take no precautions to guard against it, and of course are seldom free from it, especially the children. They imagine that it is produced by

* Lond. Med. Journal, vol. viii.
† Hist. Natural and Medic.

eating certain kinds of food, which disagree with them, from idiosyncracy; hence, some abstain from eating deers flesh, others from eating pumpkins, and some will not make use of the black pepper, uvaria piperita *, which grows spontaneously, and is very commonly used as seasoning to their food.

They cure the disease by washing with an infusion of bullanta, which is frequently not made use of until the pustules have formed large crusts, which might at first view be mistaken for yaws.

A decoction of the leaves of bellenda is also used as a lotion in this complaint. Among the Kroos, and those who live about Bassa, a plant which they call neh, achyranthes prostrata, is first dried, and then burnt; the ashes are mixed with a small quantity of water, and applied to the spots every night; it generally cures in a week, or less. A decoction of the leaves of a plant, called by the Timmanees tamba gardenia, or genippa, is sometimes used as a wash for the spots; it is a slightly acrid bitter.

A decoction of the leaves of mamunto, Timmanee, is occasionally used to wash the spots with twice a day; and for the same purpose the decoction of a plant called by the Timmanees tongamunto. The seeds of a plant called by the Timmanees akúnt, contain an oil of rather an acrid nature, which is much extolled in the cure of eruptions of the skin, intertrigo, and especially in kra-kras.

* Seu piper Æthiopicum; Tim. atchill; Bullom, neeshor.

It may not be improper to consider, as a cutaneous disease, that remarkable anomaly of the African complexion, which occurs in the albino, leucæthiops, or white negro.

Professor Blumenbach regards this curious variety of the human species as belonging to the class of diseases called cachexia ; but as this term in its more comprehensive signification implies a depraved or vitiated state of the fluids and solids of the body, incompatible with good health, it appears improper to refer it to that class; because, although this peculiarity of appearance in man, and in the lower classes of animals, such as the rabbit, weasel, and several others, be generally accompanied with debility and laxity of fibre, yet it is perfectly consistent with an healthy state of the functions. This singularity always exists previously to birth, and must of course be considered as one of the conditions of the fœtal state, which seems likely to elude the scrutiny of our limited senses.

It is supposed by Professor Sprengel * that the skin of the white negro bears a great resemblance to that of a person affected with the leprosy, an opinion which the learned author will find difficult to be maintained. It appears more probable that the Albino is the Leucæthiops of Pliny, who might be so far misled as to imagine that such a nation existed in a country so fertile in monsters as Africa †. In later times the exist-

* Handbuch der Pathologie, iii. 576.

† The same opinion is maintained by Dalin in Oratione Acad. R. Holm. " In media Africa genus hominum invenitur niveum,

ence of the Rimosses or Quimossos, a nation of dwarfs, who are said to inhabit the interior parts of Madagascar, has obtained universal belief, owing perhaps, as in the instance of the Leucæthiopians, to a solitary specimen having been produced.

This appearance of the albino is not confined to a tropical country, being frequently observable in colder regions; though it is much less striking in the white than in the black skin. Instances sometimes occur in Europe of persons who have precisely what is termed the negro cast of features, and the same peculiar appearance of the eye. Professor Blumenbach says, he has seen sixteen individuals, resembling Leucæthiopians, born in various parts of Germany.

Several instances of the white negro have fallen under my observation in Africa. In the colony of Sierra Leone there is a girl about nine or ten years of age, born in Nova Scotia, who has all the features of a negro, with woolly hair, of a dirty white colour, and whose skin equals in whiteness that of an European, without any thing disagreeable in its appearance or texture. Her eyes are between a red and light hazel

cui pili albi contortuplicati, aures longæ, palpebræ incumbentes, oculi orbiculati, iride rosea, pupillæque membrana flava, pellucida; visus lateralis in utrumque latus simul, melior tamen in tenebris quam in luce; vitæ curriculum viginti quinque annorum; corpus exiguum. Hos loqui & cogitare, terram sui causa creatam, cujus dominium se tandem obtenturos sperare." Linné Amœnitat. Acad. vol. vi. p. 74.

colour, but not much affected by the light. This may, perhaps not be considered as a proper instance, as her parents were both mulattos.

At Malacurry, in the Soosoo country, I saw a girl about the same age as the last mentioned, who was born of black parents; her skin was of an unpleasant dead looking white, and pretty smooth, though beginning to assume a cracked appearance, owing to the action of the sun. There was a man of the same colour belonging to this town, but he was then absent. This state of the skin is called by the Soosoos fong-foo, and by the Bulloms and Timmanees póolee.

At Dumboya, near Wankapong, in the Soosoo country, I saw a woman, a white negro; her parents, brothers, and sisters were all black. She was married to a black man, and had a black child. Her appearance was extremely disgusting; her skin was remarkably coarse, and wrinkled, though she was but a young woman; it was very dry and harsh to the touch, and marked with deep furrows. As she was much exposed to the sun, her skin, especially on the back, had somewhat of a reddish tinge, or cream colour; but in parts less exposed, it was of a dirty white. Large black spots, like freckles, produced by the sun, and of the size of a pea, were thickly scattered over her skin. Her hair was of a dirty yellowish white, but woolly and crisp. Her eyes were of a light bluish colour, very weak, constantly twink-

The eye brows and eye lashes were nearly white. I was informed that a boy of a similar appearance resided in the neighbourhood. At Wankapong I saw a young man about eighteen years of age, tall, and well formed, whose father had been a white negro. This young man's mother, three brothers, and two of his sisters, were black, but one sister was white like himself. His skin, from exposure to the sun, had acquired a slight reddish tinge, and was covered with a great number of black or brown spots, like freckles, some of which were nearly as large as a sixpence. It was much rougher and harsher to the touch than the woman's, feeling almost like the skin of a lizard. He complained very much of the action of the sun, which cracked his skin, and sometimes occasioned it to bleed. He was also peculiarly sensible to the bites of insects. His hair was of a dirty white, and woolly; the iris of the eye was of a reddish brown colour, and his sight very weak.

At Bottoe, on the Kroo Coast, I saw another appearance of this kind in a man about twenty-five years of age. His parents were black, and had several black children, but they had two white ones, himself and a sister. The man was very tall, rather robust, but awkward in his gait. His skin was nearly of a cream colour, and freckled from exposure, but so very much unlike that of European sailors, who expose them-

selves without shirts to the sun, that the difference was very striking at some distance. His
eyes were of a reddish colour, and very weak,
appearing red round the edges of the tarsi,
and constantly winking in a strong light. His
skin was uncommonly coarse in its texture, and
the sebaceous glands were very large and numerous. He was married to a black woman, but
had no children; his sister, whom I did not see,
was married to a black man, and had two black
children. A person informed me that he had
seen two white negroes in the Mandingo country.
In both of them, the iris was of a light blue colour; the eyes were very weak, and unable to
support the light of the sun; the hair was woolly,
and white. The skin, when closely examined,
appeared to have red patches here and there;
it was of a very coarse texture, rough, and unpleasant to the touch.

The natives consider this as a great deformity,
and look upon it as a misfortune to their family.
None of these people appeared to labour under
any imbecility of intellect. A case occurred to
me of what may be regarded as an intermediate
step to this disease: it was that of a man, of a
mulatto complexion, and much freckled, though
born of *black* parents, who had strong red hair, disposed in very small wiry curls over his whole
head. Professor Blumenbach mentions an instance of a mulatto with red hair, and quotes Von-

der Gröben *, who saw some mulattoes at Sierra Leone with this kind of hair. The pye bald negro lately exhibited at Exeter Change, London, may perhaps be referred to the same head.

An ingenious writer considers the Albinos merely as a variety of that dreadful malady called Cretinism, which occurs so frequently in the Lower Vallais, a county of Switzerland, and which is confined to a district of about thirty miles in length, and eight in breadth. The Cretins are said by this author to be " a set of beings, above indeed the brute species, but in every respect below their own. Some have a sort of voice, but the deaf and dumb are very numerous; and there are multitudes who are even mere animal machines, and devoid of almost every sensation. In point of stature, four feet and a half is the standard they reach in general, and it is seldom exceeded more than a few inches. Their countenances are *pale, wan,* and *livid*; and, exclusive of other external marks of imbecility, they have the mouth very wide, and the tongue and lips uncommonly thick and large. Nature seems also to have exhausted with them all her efforts at a very early hour, and old age treads upon the heels of infancy. They die, regularly, young, and there are not any instances of their arriving at the advanced period of human life."——The same author continues, " amidst its varieties, we find the Dondos,

* Guineische Reisebeschreibnng.

or African white negroes; the Kakerlaks, or Chacrelas, of Asia; and the Blafard, or white Indian,
of the Isthmus of Darien; all of whom have some
peculiarities corresponding with those by which
the Cretin is distinguished. The Dondos are most
common at Kongo, Loango, and Angola, and
the Kakerlaks or Chacrelas in the Java islands.
The stature of the Dondos *, the Kakerlak, and
white Indian, is nearly that of the Cretin of the
Pays de Vallais, and their whole appearance an-
nounces excessive debility and weakness. The
weakness of the eye, they are all in some degree
subject to;—this is the only circumstance in
which any similarity can be traced between the
Cretin and the African white negro, for I can by
no means agree with this gentleman, that " deaf-
ness in one degree or other is peculiar to them;"
and as little do I believe that " they all die early;

* Dr. Isert saw at Whidah a milk white negro woman sent by
the king of Dahomy to the Danish governor; she was, he says,
very ugly, not above four feet high, and appeared to have been
an *abortive* production. In the Encyclopedie Methodique, Article Medecine, tome prem. p. 318, a very just opinion is given
respecting the white negro; it is there said, " Feu Mr. le Febure
des Hayes,—demontre, ou au moins paroit demontrer, par des
faits incontestables dont il s'est assuré par lui meme, que les
hommes blancs ou blafards ne sont qu'une varietè de negres;
qu'un *albinos* nait d'une regresse qui aura egalement eu des enfans du plus beau noir, & qui n'aura connu d'hommes que ceux
de sa couleur; que cette varietè ne forme nulle part une peuple,
n'a, du cotè des sens, qu'une delicatesse que l'exercice dissipe,
n'a point une stature inferieure a celle des autres negres, & n'est
inferieur à aucun d'eux par l'intelligence, la capacitè, les qualitès
du cœur, l'aptitude au travail : il en a vu de fort agés.

and they have all the same scanty portion of intelligence."

When black people receive any considerable injury to their skin from wounds, burns, &c. the cicatrix remains white through life. It is not uncommon to see persons whose skins have undergone a change from black to white, the appearance being confined to only a small part of the body. Sometimes one or both hands and feet are spotted black and white; sometimes they are entirely white. The Bulloms compare this disease to a caterpillar, variegated black and white, which they call unnáh, and hence they name the disease ker'unnah, or spotted worm. This change of colour is not produced by any injury done to the skin. The natives appear ignorant of the cause of this curious phænomenon: some blame particular kinds of food, as they do in kra-kra, while others more prudently confess their ignorance. Dr. Isert saw a negro whose hands and feet were perfectly white, a change which had succeeded a severe illness*. Dr. Clark, of Dominica, takes notice of this curious appearance, and ascribes it to the eating of poisonous fish. " This fish poison, he says, seldom destroys life entirely, except the deadly poison of the yellow billed sprat, as it is called, which kills very speedily; but those who have eaten of the other kinds of poisonous fish are frequently reduced to the last extremity by the vomiting,

---

* Reise nach Guinea, 175.

and life is almost extinguished before stimulants*
can take effect."

" A singular effect of fish poison is to remove
the epidermiss in patches or spots, about the
hands and feet, which continue white in people
of colour, and of a pale yellow colour in white
people, for life †."

Nostalgia, maladie du pays, or an ardent desire to revisit one's native home, is a disease which
affects the natives of Africa as strongly as it
does those of Switzerland ; it is even more violent in its effects on the Africans, and often
impels them to dreadful acts of suicide. Sometimes it plunges them into a deep and incurable
melancholy, which induces the unhappy sufferers
to end a miserable existence by a more tedious,
though equally certain method, that. of dirt
eating, the effects of which will be noticed here-
after. No reader of sensibility can peruse without
emotion Haller's empassioned regret for the calm
retreat of Hasel ‡ ; but even Haller's glowing language appears cold and lifeless, if compared with
the agonizing expressions of distress poured out
by the poor African, when, waking from the sleep
in which delusive fancy had wafted him back
to his friends and much loved home, he finds only
the cruel mockery of a dream. This disease has
been supposed to be almost peculiar to the natives
of mountainous countries ; hence the Highlanders

* The poisonous effects of fish are best counteracted by the
use of capsicum.
† Med. Facts, vol. vii.   ‡ Sehnsucht nach dem Vaterlande

of Scotland, as well as the Swiss, have been remarked to be extremely prone to it. May it
not rather be said to prevail most among those
people who live in that happy state of simplicity which nature, as her choicest gift, has bestowed upon her favourites, and of which too
many have been deprived by the baneful effects
of luxury ?

CHAP. X.

GENERAL DISEASES.

BITE OF SNAKES.　OF SCORPIONS.　OF TARANTULAS.

SNAKES are so very numerous in Africa that they enter dwelling houses, and conceal themselves under beds, in pursuit of rats, lizards, cockroaches, &c. Those of the larger kind frequently make great havoc among poultry, and swallow young chickens, and even fowls of a large size *. Notwithstanding the frequent visits of these reptiles in houses, it is very rare that any fatal accidents happen, as they carefully avoid the sight of the human species †, and never bite but in self defence. No instance occurred, during my residence in the country, of any one

* The snakes have a formidable enemy in a species of ants, not larger than those in England, and from their colour called black ants. These frequently enter houses in such incredible multitudes as to cover the walls and floors, which they never quit unless driven out by fire or boiling water, until they have searched every cranny, and have destroyed every thing which has life, or which can serve them for food. Were they to find a person confined to bed by sickness, he would quickly be destroyed if not immediately removed. When they depart, the house is left perfectly desert : neither snake, rat, lizard, frog, centipes, cockroach, nor spider, the usual guests in an African hut, are to be seen.

† Lieut. Paterson gives an instance of a snake pursuing two boys, who, perhaps, had been irritating it.—Voyage to the Cape of Good Hope.

having been injured by a snake. Lieutenant
Matthews saw a boy on the island of Bananas,
who was bitten by a small black snake about four
or five feet long, and who died within two hours
after having received the wound. Nothing could
be observed in the wounded part but two small
punctures, without any appearance of inflammation*. The most poisonous species of snakes
about Sierra Leone are the following. 1. A snake
called by the Bulloms rhea, by the Timmanees
rangree, and by the Soosoos cùsse; it is about
six feet long, the head and tail inclining to red.
It is always seen on trees, and never on the ground,
its bite is considered as speedily fatal, and is
much dreaded. 2. A small, slender, green snake,
beautifully variegated with black, whose bite is
speedily mortal; it is called by the Timmanees
agboog. 3. A snake, called by the Timmanees
roff, by the Bulloms rimba, and by the Soosoos
tambaloombee, is about two feet long, and of a
darkish green colour speckled with black; its
bite is fatal. 4. Another snake, whose bite proves
fatal, is called by the Bulloms loolio, and by the
Timmanees yanketa; it is of a light grey colour,
somewhat resembling a piece of dry stick covered
with lichen, for which it is sometimes unfortunately mistaken, and handled by children.

Mr. Matthews speaks of a snake, called by the
Timmanees sinyacki-amoofong†, which is of a

* Voyage to Sierra Leone, p. 43.
† This signifies only " a bad snake."

pale green colour, with black spots; it is about a foot long, and as thick as a man's little finger. This snake is said to eject a subtile vapour to the distance of two or three feet, into the eyes of animals, which occasions extreme pain for eight or ten days, and incurable blindness. Mr. Matthews has seen several people who had suffered from this cause. This snake probably resembles that mentioned by Lieutenant Patterson*, found near the Cape of Good-Hope, called the spoog-slang, or spitting-snake, which he was informed would throw its poison to the distance of several yards, and that people have been blinded in consequence of it.

There is a small snake called by the Timmanees lafott, and by the Soosoos and Mandingos fodogoee, of a brownish colour, and about a foot long. Its bite does not prove mortal, but it excites excessive pain, and a smart fever, which continues several days.

The snake, respecting whose strength and voracity such wonderful stories have been related, is found in the neighbourhood of Sierra Leone. The skin of one which I saw, measured sixteen feet and a half in length, and appeared to have been about three or four feet in circumference; and since I left the colony, a snake of this kind has been killed, which measured twenty feet in length. Mr. Matthews says he knew an instance of one being killed a few hours after it had swallowed a large goat with kid, which was taken out entire, " the

* Travels, p. 165.

bones only being broken as if they had passed through a mill." It is called by the Bulloms pay, by the Timmanees neé-rang, and by the Soosoos tennay. Its bite is not attended with danger.

The tennay is probably of the same genus as the aboma* of Surinam. Captain Stedman having shot one of these creatures, found it to measure twenty-two feet † some inches in length, and in circumference to be as thick as a boy twelve years old round the waist. The same respectable author adds, that, when full grown, it is said to be sometimes forty feet in length, and to be more than four feet in circumference. " Its colour is a greenish black on the back, a fine brownish yellow on the sides, and a dirty white under the belly, the back and sides being spotted with irregular black rings, with a pure white in the middle. Its head is broad and flat, small in proportion to the body, with a large mouth, and a double row of teeth: it has two bright prominent eyes; is covered all over with scales, some about the size of a shilling; and under the body, near the tail, armed with two strong claws like cock-spurs, to help it in seizing its prey. It is an amphibious animal, that is, it delights in low and marshy places, where it lies curled up like a rope, and concealed under moss, rotten timber, and dried leaves, to seize its prey by surprise, which from its im-

* Boa constrictor.

† Dr. Bancroft mentions one which measured " thirty-three feet some inches ; and in the largest place, near the middle, was three feet in circumference."

mense bulk it is not active enough to pursue. When hungry it will devour any animal that comes within its reach, and is indifferent whether it is a sloth, a wild boar, a stag, or even a tiger, round which having twisted itself by the help of its claws, so that the creature cannot escape, it breaks by its irresistible force every bone in the animal's body, which it then covers over with a kind of slime or slaver from its mouth, to make it slide, and at last gradually sucks it in till it disappears. After this, the aboma cannot shift its situation, on account of the great knob or knot which the swallowed prey occasions in that part of the body where it rests, till it is digested." " I have been informed," captain Stedman continues, " of negroes being devoured by this animal, and am disposed to credit the account; for should they chance to come within its reach when hungry, it would as certainly seize them as any other animal."

The account of this prodigious snake has hitherto been commonly treated as a fable; but when we have such respectable evidence of its astonishing powers, as is given by the last mentioned author, we can no longer remain in doubt. It requires indeed a large portion of faith to believe that this creature can swallow a buffalo; but supposing it to be between twenty and forty feet in length, and nearly four feet in circumference, it does not appear incredible to suppose it capable of swallowing a wild boar, particularly if the extreme dilatability of the jaws of the snake kind

be considered. I saw at Sierra Leone a snake
of the smallest kind, not thicker than a man's
little finger, which was killed in attempting to
swallow a frog nearly three times its own size.
The snake had begun, as usually, by the head,
but after many efforts, finding it too large,
had endeavoured to reject it; these efforts were
counteracted by the frog, which pressed forwards to
escape the pressure of its enemy's jaws, and in
this state they both expired. This great extensi-
bility of the jaws of the snake is also mentioned
by the same amusing writer, in describing a
curious contest which he witnessed between a
a large frog and a snake. " When I first perceived
the frog", says captain Stedman, " his head and
shoulders were already in the jaws of the snake,
which last appeared to me about the size of a
large kitchen poker, and had its tail twisted round
a tough limb of the mangrove*; while the frog,
who appeared to be the size of a man's fist, had
laid hold of a twig, with the claws of its hinder
legs, as with hands. In this position were they
contending, the one for life, the other for his
dinner, forming one straight line between the two
branches, and thus I beheld them for some time,
apparently stationary and without a struggle.
Still I was not without hope that the poor frog
might extricate himself by his exertions, but the
reverse was the case, for the jaws of the snake gra-

---

* For an instance of frogs frequently taking up their abode in
trees, see Philosophical Transactions, vol. lxvi.

dually relaxing, and by their elasticity forming an incredible orifice, the body and forelegs of the frog by little and little disappeared, till finally nothing more was seen than the hinder feet and claws, which were at last disengaged from the twig, and the poor creature was swallowed whole by suction down the throat of his formidable adversary, whence he was drawn some inches farther down the alimentary canal, and at last stuck, forming a knob or knot at least six times as thick as the snake, whose jaws and throat immediately contracted, and re-assumed their former natural shape. The snake being out of our reach, we could not kill him, as we wished to do, to take a further examination. Thus we left him continuing in the same attitude, without moving, and twisted round the branch."

When any person has been bitten by a snake, he immediately applies a tight ligature above the wounded part; another person applies his mouth to the wound to suck out the poison, but they imagine that he must also have a grig-gree to counteract its bad effects: all this, it may be supposed, is done by a certain description of people. The wound is then scarified deeply, and is suffered to bleed: afterwards an ointment is applied, which they generally have in readiness. This is composed of the leaves of a plant called by the Soosoos lakkasai, and by the Timmanees ness; also of a plant called by the Soosoos santai, by the Timmanees apunto-kelle, and by the Bulloms issumpellen;

together with a plant called by the Soosoos tolinghe, by the Bulloms yèker, and by the Timmanees attar. Equal parts of these leaves are burnt, and the ashes are mixed into an ointment with palm oil.

They also provoke sneezing, which they consider as a favourable symptom; and to evacuate, as they suppose, the poison more completely, they endeavour to excite vomiting. These applications are all attended with a number of magical ceremonies.

The seeds of the musk plant *, hibiscus albemoschus, yield an oil, which, when taken internally, is esteemed in Guiana a specific for the bites of poisonous snakes; or a cataplasm is applied to the wound, composed of the meal of the seeds of the musk plant, or of the wild ochra, mixed with olive oil. Dr. Bancroft has seen this used with success. The same author says, the general remedy for the bites of poisonous animals is a cataplasm of the pulp of lemons or limes mixed with sea salt, and applied to the wounded part; this has frequently been found of use when the part had been previously scarified †.

Captain Carver ‡ speaks of salt as an effectual remedy against the bite of a rattle-snake; " if ap-

---

* The musky seeds of the hibiscus used formerly to be sent in large quantities from the West Indies to France; for what purpose is uncertain, but probably as a perfume. This plant is called by the Bulloms oo-feng-feng, and by the Timmanees ka-feng-feng. They burn the whole plant, mix the ashes with palm oil, and give it internally to those who have been bitten by a snake.

† History of Guiana.   ‡ Travels in North America.

plied immediately to the part, or the wound be washed with brine, a cure," he observes, " might be assured." Another remedy is mentioned by the same writer, called the rattlesnake plantain, the leaves of which chewed, and applied immediately to the wound, swallowing also some of the juice, seldom fails of proving effectual. He further adds, " so convinced are the Indians of the power of this infallible antidote, that for a trifling bribe of spirituous liquor they will at any time permit a rattle-snake to drive his fangs into their flesh." Professor Thunberg informs us, that at the Cape of Good-Hope, the blood of the turtle is greatly celebrated as an antidote against the bites of snakes, and that it is dried, and carried by every one who travels: " Whenever any one is wounded by a serpent, he takes a couple of pinches of the dried blood internally, and applies a little of it to the wound." In another part he adds, " the Hottentots, when bitten by a serpent, go in search of a toad, with which they rub the wound, and thus effect a perfect cure. They have also the art of extracting the poison, by causing another person to apply his mouth to the wound, and suck it, after scarifying the flesh all round with a knife."

A curious circumstance occurred in the River Camarancas, near Sierra Leone, which may perhaps explain how many of the supposed antidotes and infallible remedies have acquired their reputation. Two snakes of a poisonous kind were observed fighting, and one of them having been wounded, went immediately to a plant, from

whence it bit part of a leaf and instantly retired.
The natives, who witnessed the scene, brought
the remaining part of the leaf to Dr. Afzelius.

Notwithstanding the great variety of specific
remedies so much boasted of against the bites of
the most poisonous snakes, it seems probable that
the opinion of Celsus is just, who asserts that the
bites of different serpents do not require very different modes of cure. It is worthy likewise of
observation, how nearly the mode of treatment he
recommends agrees with that practised by the
Africans; in both instances the chief dependance
appears to be placed upon tight ligatures, scarifi-
cation of the wound, and sucking it by the mouth*
or by cupping-glasses.

The Africans express the strongest symptoms
of terror at the sight of these poisonous snakes,
and can scarcely be prevailed upon to touch them
even when dead. The " Psylli, Marsique, & qui
Ophiogenes vocantur," are not to be met with
upon the western coast of Africa, and their art, if
ever practised there, is now totally forgotten. It
is however still practised in some of the interior
parts of this continent, and the following curious
account of it is given by a learned and ingenious
traveller. " I can myself vouch, that all the black

* Si neque qui exsugat, neque cucurbitula, est, sorbere oportet
jus anserinum vel vitulinum, & vomere. Celsus, l. v. c. 27.

For a beautiful description of the sucking of a wound occasioned by the sting of a bee, see the Aminta of Tasso, scena seconda,
atto primo.

people in the kingdom of Senaar, whether Funge
or Nuba, are perfectly armed against the bite of
either scorpion or viper. They take the cerastes,
(a viper whose bite is mortal) in their hands at all
times, put them in their bosoms, and throw them
to one another as children do apples or balls,
without having irritated them by this usage so
much as to bite. The Arabs have not this secret
naturally, but from their infancy they acquire an
exemption from the mortal consequences attending the bite of these animals, by chewing a certain
root, and washing themselves (it is not anointing)
with an infusion of certain plants in water." He
elsewhere continues, " I have constantly observed,
that however lively the viper was before, upon
being seized by any of these barbarians he seemed
as if taken with sickness and feebleness, frequently
shut his eyes, and never turned his mouth towards
the arm of the person that held him." " They all
knew how to prepare any person by medicines,
which were decoctions of herbs and roots." " I
have seen many thus armed for a season do pretty
much the same feats as those that possessed the
exemption naturally*.

* Bruce's Travels.—Dr. Hasselquist (Voyages in the Levant,
p. 63.) gives a similar account of the Psylli in Egypt, and speaks
of a woman whom he saw handling the most poisonous and
dreadful snakes, alive and brisk, with as much unconcern as
our ladies do their laces. He adds, the art of fascinating serpents
is a secret among the Egyptians. It is known only to certain
families, who transmit it to their offspring; and the person who
fascinates serpents, never meddles with other poisonous animals,
such as scorpions, lizards, &c. The Psalmist takes notice of this

A belief in the reality of this art was generally prevalent among the ancients, but so much blended with popular superstitions, some of which are noticed by Pliny, as must have diminished its credibility. There is no doubt, that in many instances the handling of these poisonous serpents was attended with some deception; for either their bite was not effective, or if so, their fangs had been previously extracted. Celsus appears to have been one of those who bestowed no credit upon the art or its professors, he says, " Nequehercule scientiam præcipuam habent hi, qui Psylli nominantur ; sed *audaciam* usu ipso confirmatam. Nam venenum serpentis, ut quædam etiam venatoria venena quibus Galli præcipue utuntur, non gustu, sed in vulnere nocent *. Ideoque colubra ipsa tuto estur :

art (Psal. lviii. 4, 5.) when he compares the wicked to the " deaf adder that stoppeth her ear ; which will not hearken to the voice of charmers, charming never so wisely." In the Amœnit. Acad. it is said, " Certe D. D. Jacquin, ex India occidentali redux, artem excantandi serpentes sese auro redemisse, in literis ad D. Præsidem testatur: an hoc fiat masticando aristolochiam anguicidam ejusdem, vel alia methodo, nobis etiamnum latet, sed speravimus brevi hoc arcanum communicaturum cum publico D. D. Jacquin, quod avide nobiscum omnes curiosi exoptant & precibus efflagitant." xi. 216. According to Mr. Forskal, the Egyptians use for this purpose a species of aristolochia.

* Cato proceeds upon the same principle when he thus harangues his soldiers:

——————Vana specie conterrite leti
Ne dubita miles tutos haurire liquores :
Noxia serpentum est admixto sanguine pestis :
Morsu virus habent, & fatum in dente minantur :
Pocula morte carent, dixit, dubiumque venenum
Hausit.   Lucani Phars. ix. ver, 162.

ictus ejus occidit, &, si *stupente ea* (quod per
quædam medicamenta circulatores faciunt) in os
digitum quis indidit, neque percussus est, nulla in
ejus saliva noxa est. Ergo quisquis, exemplum
psylli secutus, id vulnus exsuxerit, & ipse tutus
erit, & tutum hominem præstabit. Illud interea
ante debebit attendere, ne quod in gingivis, pala-
tove, aliave parte oris ulcus habeat." If this
opinion of Celsus be just, that the whole art of
handling serpents with impunity consists in a certain degree of confidence to be acquired only
by practice, it may explain why the secret has
been confined for upwards of two thousand years
to a peculiar race of people. We know that in
England, rat-catchers handle these animals without dread, and ascribe this power to some medicine with which they anoint their hands; but their
whole secret consists in this, that they never touch
a rat until confinement and hunger have abated
his fierceness, and even then, only with the greatest
gentleness.

There are also insects in Africa of a poisonous nature, whose bites, though not attended
with fatal effects, are productive of excruciating
pain. The scorpion * is called by the Timmanees

And in like manner " Cozzi, viper-catcher to the grand duke of
Tuscany, swallowed a drachm of the poison of the viper, without
being incommoded by it, although one or two drops of it were sufficient to kill an animal when dropped into a wound." Lond.
Med. Journal, vol. i.

* The sting of the black or rock scorpion is said by Lieutenant
Patterson to be nearly as poisonous as any of the serpent tribe ;
he adds, that a farmer near the Cape of Good-Hope, who was

kooliss, by the Bulloms kelkalum, by the Soosoos
and Mandingos boontállee, and by the Foolas
yáree. It is a common observation, that children
are seldom bitten by this reptile, because it seldom quits its concealment until the evening,
when they are asleep. The scorpion is found in
great numbers, under large stones, &c. where
it takes up its abode during the day. The tarantula, as it is improperly named by the English,
aranea avicularia, is called by the Bulloms wook,
and by the Timmanees attoppur. The bite of this
insect causes more violent pain than the sting of
the preceding one, and often produces cold sweats
and fainting; but there is seldom much swelling of
the part. The practice of the natives is somewhat
inert, and patience seems to be their chief remedy.
They usually apply a tight ligature round the
limb, and rub the wound with tobacco ashes. Or
they sometimes bruise the animal* which has
inflicted the wound, burn it, and rub the ashes over
the affected part. The part is sometimes fo-
mented with a hot infusion of the leaves of the
ananas in water; or slices of the fruit are applied,
and frequently renewed.

Bites from these poisonous insects very rarely occur here, notwithstanding their great numbers,
because the inhabitants are constantly on their

stung by one of these scorpions in the foot, died within a few hours
after receiving the injury. The centipes, scolopendra morsitans,
is very common at Sierra Leone, but I never knew an accident
from it.

* Nam scorpio ipse sibi pulcherrimum medicamentum est.
Celsus, l. v. c. 27.

guard. No person will put on a pair of boots or shoes, which have not been worn for some time, without first having carefully examined whether a scorp on, tarantula, &c, be within. They are frequently introduced on board ships in the fire-wood. A black woman, about forty years of age, and very corpulent, was bitten by a tarantula between the forefinger and thumb whilst gathering some sticks. She immediately complained of a most excruciating pain running up the whole inner side of the arm to the shoulder. Her arm felt extremely cold, her whole body was covered with a cold sweat, she experienced great anxiety and oppression at her breast, and frequently fainted. Her pulse was so very small and creeping, as scarcely to be felt at the wrist. She took three grains of pure opium immediately, and her arm was fomented with a decoction of three ounces of camomile flowers in two pounds of water, in which were dissolved three drachms of crude opium. The fomentation was continued near two hours without producing the smallest abatement of the pain ; it appeared, indeed, rather to increase in violence. The fainting fits became more frequent and were of longer continuance. She complained of universal coldness, her hand felt cold to the touch, and seemed to her to have lost all sensation. The whole arm was affected with very acute pain, especially when touched. The pain was greatly aggravated at intervals, and produced frequent and severe rigors. A considerable degree of tightness soon extended over the muscles of the breast, and produced much uneasiness and difficulty in respiration. The fomentations were ordered to be very frequently repeated; she swallowed again three grains of opium, and took a scruple of camphor dissolved in an ounce of water. In about an hour after having taken the draught, she felt the pain rather easier, and it was then entirely confined to the arm. The tightness and difficulty of respiration had entirely ceased. Her pulse became fuller, and beat about seventy strokes in a minute. The skin was also warm, and a general moisture began to break out. Towards evening the pain had almost wholly disappeared, and she could bear her arm to be touched. Next day she had no other complaint than a degree of languor.

Very excruciating pain is frequently produced by a wound from the sting-ray, pastinaca marina. A black man, about fifty years of age, whilst fishing, was wounded by a sting-ray upon the anterior part of the tibia, about two inches above the malleolus internus. Much blood was discharged from the wound, and he was obliged to be carried home. The pain was so exquisite, that he could not continue a moment in one posture; his pulse beat only sixty times in a minute, and was very small, and intermitted every fourth stroke. A cold clammy sweat covered his whole body. The wound appeared to be pretty smoothly cut, and was about a quarter of an inch in length. From the wound to the foot he had no other sensation than that of extreme coldness. Above the wound, the pain was so very acute along the inner side of the leg to the knee, that he could not bear upon it the slightest pressure. No hardness could be felt in the course of the lymphàtics, and over the wound there was only a slight elevation, scarcely percepti-ble, and rather hard. He was affected at intervals with such severe rigors as shook his whole frame. Three grains of pure opium were immediately exhibited. In an hour after having taken the opium, he felt not the least abatement of pain; his pulse still continued slow and intermitting, but was rather fuller. The rigors were as severe as before, and his face was covered with a cold clammy sweat. The part was ordered to be fo-mented, as in the last case, for ten minutes, and then to be covered with a liniment composed of a drachm of opium and the same quantity of camphor dissolved in a little spirit, and then rub-bed up with an ounce of oil: a draught was also given, composed of fifteen grains of camphor, and forty drops of tincture of opium. After this had been taken, and the fomentations applied the se-cond time, the pain abated considerably, and the rigors entirely left him. The pulse had now in-creased to seventy beats in a minute, and was regu-lar and full. Upon touching the wound, or the inner surface of the leg, he still complained of ex-quisite pain. The fomentations were ordered to be continued, and in about five hours from the acci-dent he was perfectly easy, except when the part was touched.

CHAP. XI.

GENERAL DISEASES.

BURNS AND SCALDS. ULCERS. RECENT WOUNDS. FRACTURES.

IN some cases of BURNS and SCALDS, the Africans beat up the egg of a fowl, and rub it upon the part, applying over it fine cotton, which is permitted to remain until it drop off: in other cases, the part is rubbed with palm oil. The cold pulp of the calibash is also applied as a cataplasm, and frequently renewed. Among the Kroos, the vesication is opened and the skin removed; after which the ashes of the leaves of obiss are applied to the part.

ULCERS, called by the Bulloms oo-pa, or oo-pil, by the Timmanees kissam, or ka-pil, constitute a very extensive and troublesome class of diseases in Africa. They may be produced by the most trifling causes, as the bite of a muskito, or a slight scratch of the skin, and become often so inveterate as to resist every mode of treatment. In warm climates, the body acquires a morbid degree of irritability, highly unfavourable to the healing of ulcers, and which occasions them to spread rapidly. This is experienced as well by the natives, as by European sailors, who, following their example, go without shoes, and are thus rendered liable to accidents on the lower extremities, which lay the foundation for incurable maladies.

The applications made use of by the natives are of an astringent quality, and consist principally of barks of trees. Decoctions of these are used as washes: sometimes the bark in a coarse powder is sprinkled over the surface of the ulcer; or it is formed into an ointment with palm oil. Some degree of pain is usually excited by these applications, many of which are of a very stimulant and active nature. No bandages are applied, and the patients are allowed to use as much exercise as they are able. At every dressing, which is seldom repeated more than once a day, the surface of the sore is washed perfectly clean. It does not appear to me, from the general success, that any of these applications is possessed of a specific power. I have seen instances where the natives have cured ulcers which had baffled all the attempts of Europeans; and I have seen the same success attend the European mode of dressing, where the natives had been unsuccessful: I have also seen cases which foiled both modes of cure. As the applications of the natives are of a stimulant nature, sometimes violent in their operation, and used in all cases indiscriminately, without regard to the state of the ulcer, or the health of the patient, it often happens that in irritable habits they cause ulcers to spread considerably, and become sloughy; but in cases where there is a want of action in the part, they generally succeed. Sometimes the healing process goes on remarkably well for a few days, after which the sore relapses into its former state, or becomes worse. The sudden amendment above mentioned in the appearance of ulcers, seems not to depend upon any kind of difference in the application, but rather upon a proper degree of stimulus casually used. Among the various applications to ulcers, the following are in most repute. A decoction of the leaves of bullanta is used as a wash for ulcers when foul and sloughy: it is a powerful astringent, and gives some pain when applied. This tree has been already noticed for its virtues: the pith of the smaller branches is chewed in order to heal scorbutic ulcers of the mouth; it is also used to clean the mouth when foul; in its operation it produces a copious discharge of saliva. In the West Indies the fresh root of the bitter cassada is frequently scraped, and applied to ill-conditioned ulcers. At Sierra Leone the sweet cassada is boiled and beaten until it become smooth; it is then applied warm as a poultice; its good effects appear wholly to result from the heat and moisture communicated.

The bark of a tree, called by the Bulloms bongiare, and by the Timmanees pongia cananga, may be considered as the most popular remedy for ulcers. It is a strong and rather unpleasant bitter, but has very little astringency. When chewed, or infused in water, it readily yields a beautiful and durable yellow colour, which is used by the natives for dying mats, &c. The powder of this bark is sprinkled upon the ulcer every day, and if the sore be large, it is applied twice a day; but when there appears a disposition to heal, the application is made but once a day. A decoction of this bark is also used as a wash to the ulcer previously to the use of the powder. When the powder has been applied two or three days, a crust forms round the edge of the sore, and is pulled off when dry.

Bungaroo is a species of vine, so called by the Bulloms and Timmanees, and employed by them to fasten the rafters of their houses. It is cut into small pieces, and boiled in water for a considerable time. This decoction is used warm, and applied every day to ulcers in which there is much sloughing: when the slough is removed, the surface of the ulcer is covered with the fine scrapings of the following.

'N-koot, Bullom; támmaree, Soosoo; mabait, Timmanee; elate sylvestris. This is a plant of the palm kind, bearing a small red fruit, which the natives eat. The stem of the plant, when deprived of its outer skin, is scraped into a very light, down-like substance, resembling fine wool or cotton. It is applied to ulcers after they are washed, with the same view as lint, to absorb the purulent matter: it is remarkably soft, and is laid over the surface of the sore, to the thickness of half an inch; it adheres of itself, without being confined by any bandage. I saw this used by a young man, about twenty years of age, who had been afflicted from childhood with scrophulous complaints. He had, when I saw him, a very extensive ulcer affecting the elbow. It was cellular like an honeycomb, and several sinuses seemed to run toward the joints. The surface of the sore was clean, but covered with florid, loose, spongy granulations. He had lost the use of both elbow joints, and the diseased arm was much wasted above the elbow. This case appeared to be chiefly left to nature, as no other application was made use of but the scrapings of mabait, which were renewed every morning : they adhered much closer than lint, and could not be removed until well soaked in a warm decoction of the same wood. This decoction has no sensible qualities. He had followed this plan of treatment about two months, with little apparent benefit. In the same town were two women, who had the scars of scrophulous ulcers, one under the angle of the lower jaw, the other over the sternum.

When an ulcer becomes foul, or the flesh begins to rise too high, they sometimes sprinkle it with the rust scraped from a brass pan : this practice they have probably learnt from Europeans.

The root of makunt, Timmanee; continghee, Bullom, are boiled in water, and the decoction is employed to wash ulcers. A mixture of lime juice and iron rust, of the consistence of pap, is much recommended for the cure of ulcers, and is repeated every day. The pulp of roasted limes is likewise applied, but excites much pain, and often causes the sore to spread. Dr. Wright, of

Jamaica, recommends the pulp of roasted oranges as a poultice, which, he says, corrects the fætor within twenty-four hours, and disposes the ulcer to heal soon : this application must be continued until the sore be healed*.

A decoction of the bark of léligunt, Timmanee; púlpellee, Bullom ; connarus Africanus, is used as a wash.

The leaves of two plants, called by the Soosoos korass-wurree and tansai, are made into a kind of paste with water, and applied to ulcers.

A decoction of the leaves of makoot-a-koot, Timmanee, somewhat acrid to the taste, is used as a wash for ulcers.

A decoction of the fruit of baalay, Timmanee, is used in the same manner, though it has no sensible qualities.

The bark of mekkamakengee, or " sweet substance," reduced to powder, and boiled in palm oil, is used as an application to ulcers. It is applied only every second day, and is washed off by a decoction of the leaves of the same plant. This dressing excites pain, but of no long continuance : when chewed it imparts a sweetish acid taste, and after some time leaves a sensation of astringency and acrimony, though not very strong.

The bark of tokakelle, Soosoo; messer-a-toke, fowl's egg, Timmanee, is scraped very fine and mixed with palm oil, to be applied as a dressing. The leaves of the same plant bruised, and infused

* Lond. Med. Journal, vol. viii.

in water, are much celebrated among the Kroos as a styptic, and particularly recommended in gun shot wounds. The bark of the locust tree, called by the Soosoos náyree, is dried, and reduced to a fine powder, which, mixed with palm oil, is applied warm to obstinate ulcers.

Among the Kroos, a leaf of a plant called by them gheang, and by the Timmanees apell, is frequently applied to ulcers. The young leaves, when just appearing, are dried and powdered, and sprinkled over the sore, after it has been previously washed with a decoction of a plant, called by the Kroos sassara-winghee. The leaves of apell come out in pairs, as it were glued together, and afterwards expand. They are plucked for use before they have separated, from a superstitious fear lest a hole should be made in the ulcer. These leaves have a rough and astringent taste. The Timmanees employ a decoction of the leaves of this plant to wash ulcers, especially those of the toes.

The leaves of the amelliky are used by the people about Bassa, on the Grain Coast, in the cure of ulcers. The young leaves, after being moistened in water, are wrapped in a piece of plantain leaf, and laid upon hot ashes; when thoroughly warmed, they are taken out, and their juice is pressed out upon the sore, which is then covered with a piece of plantain leaf made hot in the fire: the juice is of a brownish colour, of a slightly acid and astringent taste. I saw it effectual in a small, obstinate, ill-looking ulcer, which had resisted every other application. A popular remedy somewhat similar to the above, is used by the poor in some parts of Ireland for the cure of scrophulous ulcers. It is composed of the leaves and stalks of wood-sorrel, (oxalis acetosella) and the root of meadow sweet, (spiræa ulmaria). " The sorrel is prepared by wrapping it in a cabbage leaf and macerating it by its own juices in warm peat ashes. This pulp is applied as a poultice to the ulcer, and left twenty-four hours; the application of sorrel is four times repeated; then the roots of the meadow sweet, bruised and mixed with the sour-head or efflorescence that appears on butter-milk left in the churn, are used in the same manner till the sore heals, which always speedily happens, often in two or three weeks." Beddoes on the medical Use and Production of Factitious Airs, p. 47.

The plantain leaf, according to Atkins*, " is an admirable detergent in foul, sanious ulcers, stripped of the inner skin, and applied as you do houseleek in corns." It is frequently applied by Europeans as a dressing for blisters, which purpose it answers remarkably well. The natives usually spread their poultices upon a plantain leaf.

In FRESH WOUNDS, to restrain the hæmorrhage, they use the juice expressed from the fruit of the unripe plantain, with which they wash the wound. Among the Bulloms, a young banana tree is cut down and well heated over the fire, and the hot juice squeezed upon the wound. The medical virtues of this plant are noticed in the Encyclopedia Methodique, where it is said, " selon Min-

* Voyage to Guinea.

guet, l'eau du corps ou du tronc de la plante, est bonne pour les cours de ventre, pour nettoyer les yeux. Celle des boutons convient pour deterger les ulcères. L'ecorce du fruit vert, reduite en charbons ou pulverisée, guerit les ulceres & les crables ou fentes qui viennent sous la plante des pieds des negres. La banane jouit de la vertu aphrodisiaque." Tom. III. p. 586. Sometimes they bruise the leaves of the cotton tree, and heat them over the fire, after which the juice is pressed out upon the wound : it has an astringent taste. The flowers of the cotton shrub folded in its leaves, and roasted over the fire, yield a reddish oily liquor, which has been much commended for the cure of old ulcers. The seeds of the cotton shrub, are said to intoxicate parrots and parroquets. No other mode of restraining the flow of blood is practised than by the application of these and such like astringents. Wounds of the large vessels, above the elbow or knee, are considered as certainly fatal, but when they happen below these parts, it is thought the patient may recover. Theft is punished among the Foolas by dividing the tendo achillis and the surrounding muscles to the bone: when the patient is weakened by the loss of blood, they apply to the wound a kind of actual cautery consisting of boiling wax. This is the only case that has come to my knowledge in which they use heat to restrain hæmorrhages; but according to some late travellers in Africa, it is not unfrequently employed. Mr. Lempriere says, he was informed in Morocco, "that legs and arms are taken off by a common knife and saw, and that the stump is afterwards dipped in boiling pitch, which is the only mode of stopping the hæmorrhage with which they are acquainted*. Mr. Brisson, speaking of the Arabs, says, "to cure the deepest wounds they use nothing but earth." "They have another expedient to remove pains, but not so efficacious, applying a red hot iron to the part affected." Mr. Saugnier, speaking of a tribe of Moors called Mongearts, who live in the neighbourhood of Galam, about nine hundred miles above the mouth of the river Senegal, says, "flesh wounds are cured with fire ; that is to say, a stab is treated by cauterizing the injured part with the red hot blade of a knife. Turtles oil and tar are then put upon it, the wound is enveloped with herbs of known efficacy, and by these means they bring about a speedy cure †."

A decoction of the bark of a large tree, called by the Timmanees keeta, is applied to fresh wounds; and the application is repeated several times a day: when the wound is nearly brought to cicatrize, the wash is omitted, and the bark itself, coarsely powdered, is sprinkled upon the sore. They also use for the same purpose, and in the same manner, the bark of a tree, called by the Timmanees attár‡, and by the Bulloms yayker. The bark of an erythrina with scarlet flowers, called

* Journey to Morocco.
† Voyages to the Coast of Africa by Saugnier and Brisson.
‡ Arbor fructu ovali acidulo,

by the Bulloms and Timmanees faatee, is reduced to powder and boiled in palm oil; it is then wrapped up in a cloth, and applied warm like a cataplasm to fresh wounds: this is continued until the cure be completed. The bark of leligunt (connarus Africanus) scraped fine and mixed with palm oil, or sometimes alone, is applied to fresh wounds, to restrain the hæmorrhage.

In FRACTURES they have been successful in every instance which occurred to my notice. They first measure the sound limb with a piece of stick, and applying it to the fractured one, they use such a degree of extension as will bring it to the same length. In compound fractures they are less fortunate; they attempt to force back the protruding end of the bone, and where this cannot be done, they imagine the use of the limb to be irrecoverably lost, and attempt to heal the wound in this state. In such cases, if the patient recover, the knee, when the leg is the part injured, is bent, and the leg fastened to the thigh by a kind of bandage which passes round them both, and is further supported by a sling from the shoulders; the patient supporting himself by a stick. A case was related to me of a celebrated general of the Foolas, who had been wounded in the foot by a poisoned arrow, in consequence of which mortification came on, and the bones separated spontaneously half way up the leg; he now walks by the aid of a stick, having his leg supported in the manner above described. When the limb has been restored to its proper length, they wrap it up in cloth, having pieces of split bamboo applied at the sides by way of splints. The Mandingos, &c. rub it with some kind of ointment, and recite over it passages of the Koran; this was the practice employed in the case of an old man who had fractured his thigh by a fall from his horse, and whom my brother saw at Teembo. He was recovering very fast, and was able to sit up in bed in about a month or six weeks after the accident. In most cases of fractures, they apply a cataplasm, composed of the bark of a tree called by the Bulloms yum: this is beaten to a pretty fine powder, and is mixed with cold water to a proper consistence, and applied over the whole leg. The limb is looked at every three days.

Among the Foolas an opinion prevails respecting TWINS, similar to that respecting seventh sons in England; they imagine them capable of acquiring great medical knowledge, and that they are peculiarly fitted for the practice of surgery, more especially for the cure of fractures.

CHAP. XII.

THE DISEASES OF WOMEN,

WITH THE SEXUAL PECULIARITIES IN AFRICA.

HYSTERIA. CATAMENIA. LABOURS. EXPULSION OF
THE PLACENTA. ABORTION. MISCARRIAGE. MILK
BREASTS. PENDULOUS BELLIES. SUCKLING.

THE diseases to which women are liable upon the coast of Africa are, as may be supposed from their mode of living, much fewer than in Europe. HYSTERIA, and the whole train of nervous diseases, are totally unknown among them. Atkins observes, " Whydah slaves are more subject to small pox, and sore eyes; other parts, to a sleepy distemper; and to windward, exomphaloses. There are few instances of deformity any where. Even their nobles know nothing of chronical distempers, nor their ladies of the vapours." Women even appear to enjoy, upon the whole, a greater immunity from sickness than the men, probably owing to their greater temperance and more active life.

The CATAMENIA occur at an early period, but to judge from appearances, probably not before the twelfth year. The quantity is nearly the same as in Europe; but the African are not liable to the same irregularities as European women The continuance of the discharge is from two to four days. It is so generally thought to be produced by the influence of the moon, that it receives its name from this planet along the whole of the windward coast. The Mandingos call it karro, or the moon; the Soosoos call it kaykay, the moon; and the Timmanee women, at its periodical return, say, the moon has caught them. The discharge itself is called by the Timmanees mateer, blood: the Mandingos call it yelissee, and use the term woollee to express blood, whether venous or arterial.

They entertain the erroneous notions respecting the noxious qualities of the catamenia, which were so universally prevalent in Europe at the commencement of the foregoing century* ; and they suppose meat would immediately become corrupted by being touched by a woman in this state. Upon some parts of the Gold Coast, women under these circumstances are not permitted to touch a man; and at Whydah they dare not at

* These idle notions are thus described by the learned De Graaf, " Si novella vitis eo tangatur in perpetuum læditur, steriles fiunt tactæ fruges, moriuntur insita, exuruntur hortorum germina ; si mulier prægnans alterius menstrua supergrediatur, aut illis circumlinatur, abortum facit : ei autem quæ uterum non gestat, concipiendi spem adimet : purgantis spiritus & vapor ab ore specula atque eboris nitorem obscurat ; gustatus hic sanguis canes in rabiem agit, homines vero diris cruciatibus affligit, comitialem morbum, pilorum effluvium, aliaque elephanticorum vitia infert: idcirco à veteribus inter venena relatus, pari malignitate existimatur atque sanguinis elephantici potus." The same opinions were entertained in the time of Pliny. Hist. Nat. lib. xxviii. cap. 7, &c.

such times enter the palace of the king, or the house of a great man, under pain of death or perpetual slavery *. To give notice of their being in this situation, they usually paint their face with a streak of yellow : this is also practised upon other parts of this continent. Among the Moors called Monselemines, who inhabit Bilidulgerid, when the women paint only one side of their face, they have no communication with the men ; a custom that is common to all the Moorish nations, as far as the banks of the Niger †. About El Mina, when the catamenia first appear, the face and body are painted white, to denote that the person is marriageable. This is also the practice among the women of Chili : " Si matris sit filia aliqua matura viro, quæ tamen non petatur, tunc mater eam sub oculis rubro colore pingit, ubi menses suos semel passa fuerit ‡." The same people are said to wear their hair loose in general, but to tie it up at a certain time, viz. " quando mensibus laborant, atque hoc indicium facit."

In the Mandingo country, a menstruating woman is considered as unclean, and capable of defiling every thing she touches : during this period she resides alone in a small hut, built for the purpose, in some secluded spot, where she continues until well ; she then washes, and appears in public as usual. If women should happen to go into public in this state, they salute no person, but

* Bosman.
† Voyages to Africa by Saugnier and Brisson.
‡ Marcgrave de Brasileæ Regione, &c.

withdraw their hands, as a signal of being unclean. They cannot at these times join in the public prayers, nor cook, wash, or indeed do any thing for their husbands. This last custom prevails also among the Bulloms and Timmanees, except where the man is so poor as to have only one wife, in which case his indolence lets him allow her services at all times. Niebuhr makes the same observation, " Les Mahometanes qui ont les in-commodites de leur sexe, n'osent faire leurs prieres accoutumées, c. a. d. les Hanefites pendant dix jours & les Schafeites pendant quinze par le prin-cipe, qu'il faut etre pur quand on paroit devant Dieu. Les payennes des Indes n'osent toucher personne pendant ce temps, & tant que cette in-firmite dure, elles sont recluses dans un coin ou on leur porte ce qui leur est necessaire."

Among the Indians of America, this state of seclusion at the monthly period is very strictly observed. In every camp or town, there is an apartment appropriated, to which both single and married women retreat, and there confine them-selves till the catamenia cease : they are afterwards purified in running streams, and then return to their different employments. The men on these occasions most carefully avoid holding any communication with them ; and the Naudowessies are so rigid in this observance, that they will not suffer any belonging to them to fetch from these monthly retreats of the females, such things as are necessary, not even fire, though the want of them be attended with the greatest inconvenience.

They are further so superstitious as to think, if a pipe stem cracks, which among them is made of wood, that the possessor has either lighted it at one of these polluted fires, or held some converse with a woman during her retirement, which is esteemed by them most disgraceful and wicked*."

The women at Akra, on the Gold Coast, bury the cloth which they have worn during the menstrual period, supposing that when it begins to rot, the woman who wore it will become pregnant: for this purpose old worn out linens (schlaptucher) are sent out, particularly from Holland; from whence also they are brought by the Danes with the same view†.

Their LABOURS are in general very easy, and are trusted solely to nature; for though some old woman commonly presides, the delivery is sometimes conducted without a single attendant, or without its being known to any one, until the woman makes her appearance at the door of the hut with the child in her arms. Upon the Gold Coast, it is considered as infamous for a woman in labour to cry out. Unfortunate cases, however, occur, where, the powers of nature being ineffectual, the woman dies undelivered, her attendants being unacquainted with any means of rendering her assistance. In such cases they frequently suspend the woman by her heels to alter the position of the child, or they put her into a

* Carver's Travels in America.
† Roemer Nachricht vonder Kuste Guinea.

variety of postures, rolling her about, and rubbing the abdomen with their hands smeared with
palm oil. This subject is particularly noticed by
Dr. Schotte, in a letter to the celebrated professor
Stein, " Depuis mon sejour ici, il y en a une negresse de morte dans ses couches, ou plutot sans
accoucher : peut etre aurois je pu lui porter de se-
cours, si le prejugé general du pays ne m'en avoit
empechè, qui est de ne jamais laisser un homme
approcher une femme dans cette condition.—
Lorsque l'accouchante a eu des douleurs reiterées,
& les sages femmes ne voyent pas paroitre l'enfant,
sans s'embarasser de sa situation dont elles n'ont
pas la moindre idée, elles prennent une drap plus
long que large, font une tour autour du ventre de
l'accouchante, & une demie douzaine de femmes
tirent de chaque bout de drap de toute leur force
pour exprimer l'enfant, la negresse, dont je viens
de porter, fut tirée de la facon." In another letter
he continues, " La facilité d'enfanter des negresses
depend selon moi de la bonne conformation des os
du bassin : elles sont dans l'etat ordinaire plus re-
trecies que chez les femmes blanches ; la cause est,
je crois, l'usage de l'eau froide, dont elles se lavent
les parties a chaque instant, non pas cependant
avec cette intention, mais pour prevenir les excori-
ations & les chancres produits assez souvent sans
aucune virus venerien par la chaleur, le sejour,
l'epaissement, & l'acreté de l'humeur qui lubrifie
cettes parties*." Captain Carver mentions the case

---

* Soemmering ueber die korperliche verschiedenheit des negers
vom europaer.

of an Indian woman, who was delivered in consequence of a general convulsion, induced by stopping for a short time the mouth and nose, so as to obstruct breathing. This is the only case which Dr. Rush has found recorded of the Indians assisting nature in parturition. The effects of sudden terror are sometimes employed among the Canadians, where it is the custom, when a woman is in labour, for the young men to surround the cabin privately, and suddenly raise a great shout*. The Africans imagine that male children lie towards the right side, and females towards the left. In difficult cases, they suppose the child is drawn up towards the stomach of the mother. Among the Kroos, when a woman falls in labour, she is removed from her own house to a small one built at a little distance, where all the women of the place accompany her, and where she continues to reside until she recovers, which is from two days to a week. These people use the following superstitious mode of hastening delivery. A woman goes to some retired place, where no one can see her, in order to procure a kind of grass, which they call daing, a species of panicum ; this she takes hold of just below the panicle, with the view of pulling it, together with the peduncle, out of the vagina which incloses it. This is to be done with the greatest gentleness, for if the least noise or snap be heard, that grass is thrown away and another is taken. If

* Jeffery's History of the French Dominions in North and South America.

this come out without making a noise, it is bruised
and put into a calibash of water, and given the
woman to drink : whilst drinking it, she is obliged
to stand upright, the empty calibash is taken from
her, and carried in a straight line from her lips to
between her feet, where it is laid, which is supposed to expedite the expulsion of the child. They
are generally delivered in a recumbent posture
upon a mat laid on the ground.

When the PLACENTA is not immediately expelled after the birth of the child, they tie a string to
the end of the funis umbilicalis, and fasten it to
the woman's foot, at the same time obliging her
to retain her breath, or to blow strongly into her
hand. When this method fails, they apply a tight
bandage round the abdomen ; sometimes they
endeavour to excite vomiting or sneezing, by
tickling the fauces, or irritating the nose with a
straw. The Soosoos, in order to expel the placenta when long retained, make the woman stand
upright, and shake her; they also give her very
cold water to drink, which they suppose con-
stringes the internal parts, and causes the placenta
to separate. After it is expelled, in order to obviate the bad effects of the cold water, some warm
fowl soup, well seasoned with piper Ethiopicum, is
given to drink. Sometimes the fine powder of the
bark of tansai is mixed in cold water, and given the
woman to drink.

The placenta is called by the Timmanees opoo-
roo, and by the Soosoos lagghee. When expelled,
they put it into an old pot and bury it ; they would

shudder at the idea of burning it : were it not to be buried, they suppose the child, when it grew older, would be affected with kra-kras. Among the Mahommedans and Soosoos, the placenta is put into an earthen pot, and well covered with leaves, that no dirt may get to it before it putrefies : it is then buried, and carefully watched for forty days,* that nothing may disturb the place : at the end of this period the woman, having previously washed herself, is dressed in white, her head is also covered with a white cloth, and going to the place she prays over it ; after which any one may go there, and even dig the pot up if he please.

The time that a woman is confined to her house after delivery is various ; in the Mandingo, Soosoo, and Foola countries, it is generally seven days, after which she immediately resumes her ordinary occupations : among the Timmanees and Bulloms, it is from two days to four or six.

A Soosoo woman was delivered at Free Town, the child and placenta being expelled together. After tying † the umbilical cord, and washing the child with warm water, it was laid upon a mat

---

* By the Levitical law a lying-in woman was unclean for forty days, until the end of which period she could not approach the altar, nor enter the temple. Among the Greeks it was held as a defilement to touch a woman in this state.

† This is the custom in the neighbourhood of Sierra Leone, and the adjoining countries. In Guiana, the umbilical cord is divided by " a brand of fire," which cauterises the orifices of the vessels, and renders a ligature unnecessary. Dr. Hasselquist says, the Turks cut the navel string, and apply to it the actual cautery.

loosely covered with a piece of cloth, and no further applications were made to it. When the funis dropped off, the navel was anointed with the pow-dered bark of a tree called nintee, mixed with palm oil. The woman sat up the second day, and walked out at the end of the week. Immediately after delivery, she washed herself from head to foot with a warm decoction of the leaves of dun-dakky in water, and then anointed herself with oil. The washing with the same decoction, and anointing afterwards with oil, was repeated every morning for the space of a month: during this time she drank of a decoction of a species of grass called maylie by the Soosoos, with a view to pro-mote the lochial discharge.

The infant is not permitted to suck its mother immediately after birth, but is given to some other woman to be suckled for the first three or four days, or until the mother's breasts be quite full. The Soosoos do not permit the child to suck until the first week be passed over: they have no ob-jection to allow a child three or four months old to suck a woman lately delivered, because they suppose it strong enough to bear the purgative effects of the milk, which, in their opinion, might prove very dangerous to an infant. In general, however, the first milk is thrown away, and the breast is carefully washed before the child be applied to it, lest it be hurt, as they say, by any of the *bad* milk. Allowing the breasts to become so much distended before they are emptied, together with the practice of binding them tight with a cloth, is probably the cause of the large and pendulous breasts remarked in the women who have borne children in this country, and not the early age at which they bring forth, as some have imagined. When speaking of their eldest child, they say, " he made their breasts fall."

Attempts to procure ABORTION are, as may be supposed, much less frequent here than in Europe: in some rare instances, however, it happens that a woman, in order to conceal an illicit connection, makes use of some medicine to restore the menstrual discharge. For this purpose they usually drink a warm infusion of the grass called maylie, or with the same intention, an infusion of a plant called by the Soosoos seng-eng-yay. Dr. Bancroft says, that female slaves in Guiana, who intend to procure abortion, make use of a diet of ochras, " by which they lubricate the uterine passages, and afterwards expel their contents, usually by the sensitive plant; though in Barbadoes a vegetable called gulley-koot is commonly used for this purpose." As the okra possesses only the sensible qualities of a mucilaginous plant, it seems improbable that it can have any such effects upon the body: the natives about Sierra Leone consider it as highly nutritious, and somewhat of a restringent. In the West Indies also it constitutes a principal part of the highly nutritious pepper pot. Artificial abortion is one of those crimes which is peculiar to a state of civilization, and prevails in proportion as luxury extends its destructive empire. It was so frequent during the depraved state of manners which accompanied the decline of the Roman Empire, that Juvenal observes :

——Jacet aurato vix ulla puerpera lecto
Tantum artes hujus, tantum medicamina possunt,
Quæ steriles facit——— vi. 593.

Women who have had one or two MISCARRIAGES are ordered to drink a decoction of a plant called by the Soosoos soongee, boiled with rice : it is very rough and astringent to the taste. When a woman has miscarried two or three times successively among the Soosoos, they are of opinion that she has, at some former period of her life, trod upon the eggs of a species of goatsucker, which they call labbatanyee : to remedy this, the woman is ordered to watch one of these birds, to discover upon what tree or shrub it settles to feed, from using which as a medicine they hope to obtain a cure. This is the bird spoken of by Moore, who says, " there is here a remarkable bird, of about the size of a pigeon, which comes abroad at dusk, and has four wings *." A similar opinion is noticed by Dapper, who says, the inhabitants of Sierra Leone imagine that if they have trod upon the eggs of a bird called jouwa, all their children will die. This misfortune is remedied by the party avoiding afterwards to eat the flesh of any bird, and calling the next child jouwa, after the name of the bird which caused the spell.

* Voyage to the Gambia.

The enlargement termed MILK BREASTS sometimes are of frequent occurrence; and women who
have had children are sometimes seen having one
breast very large, pendulous, and streaming with
milk, while the other is very small, and shrivelled
up to nothing. This is owing to the small breast
having been sore, and the child in consequence
having constantly sucked the sound one. When
the breasts become much distended with milk,
and hard, the women endeavour to force out
the milk by frequent pressure; at the same time
they put on a plant called by the Timmanees
matchill, and by the Bulloms tabakoi: this is
first bruised between two stones, and then mixed
with a little water, so as to form a thick paste,
which is permitted to dry upon the breast. A
warm infusion of a plant called by the Timmanees
ok-kunt*, by the Bulloms kunt, and by the Soosoos
continghee, ximenioides or monkey apple, is used
to foment the breasts. When a woman weans
her child, in order to repel the milk, she rubs over
her neck and breasts the bark of a tree finely powdered and mixed with water, called by the Timmanees affook: it is of a sweetish acid taste, and
has a slight degree of astringency.

Large PENDULOUS BELLIES are sometimes seen
in women who have borne children: to avoid this,
which they look upon as a deformity, it is customary for them, after lying-in, to wear a kind of
wooden hoop or a tight bandage round their waist,

* In the plural ma-kunt.

for two or three weeks after they first come out.
Women who have been troubled with exomphalos,
generally lose it entirely after the first child, or
it becomes much smaller.

They suckle their children two years, or until
the child can bring the mother a calibash full of
water : during this time they avoid all connection
with their husbands*, lest the child should be made
sick, or as they say, " lest it spoil the child." When
a child dies upon the Gold Coast, they say, the
mother has either had connection with her husband, or played the whore, or the child has been
bewitched. The same practice and opinions prevail among the North American Indians.

* In the Koran it is ordered that women shall suckle their children during two entire years, if they will suck so long. Chap. 2.
This practice though in itself bad, has originated from prudential
motives ; for the mother, upon whom devolves the whole care of
the children, is afraid of being burthened with a second offspring
before the first can in some degree dispense with her continued
care.

CHAP. XIII.

THE DISEASES AND MANAGEMENT OF CHILDREN.

TREATMENT AFTER THE BIRTH. LOCKED JAW. ME-
THOD OF CARRYING CHILDREN. ERUPTIONS. IN-
DISTINCT ARTICULATION. TINEA CAPITIS. WEAK-
NESS. WASTING. DIARRHŒA. PROTRUSIONS OF
THE NAVEL. RICKETS. PROLAPSUS ANI. DIRT
EATING. LARGE BELLIES.

THE management of children in Africa is very
simple : their diseases are also few, and of no
great importance: immediately after birth, the
infant is washed in warm water, or soap and water;
this is continued for a few days, after which cold
water only is used. During very hot weather it
is usual for the mother to throw a vessel of cold
water upon the child's head two or three times
a day, apparently to the satisfaction of the latter. After the morning ablution the child is well
greased from head to foot.

Soon after a child is born, a few grains of malaguetta pepper are bruised, and tied up in a cotton rag, which is moistened with water, and the
juice of it is pressed out into the child's mouth :
this is done to evacuate the meconium. In order to strengthen a child born at the end of

seven months, the mother takes every morning a mouthful of cold water, which she spirts upon the inside of the joints of the arms, wrists, knees, and successively, those of the whole body, immediately after which the child is immersed in very cold water. This practice is repeated every morning until they suppose the child strong enough to bear the shock of cold water without any preparation.

Dr. Zimmerman has, by copying the ingenious and elegant Buffon, been led into a venial error, when he says, " the new born children of the negroes are so very sensible, that even in their hot climate they are obliged to shut them up in warm rooms for the nine first days, as they are liable to be attacked with TRISMUS from the smallest breath of external air." This is, however, so far from being the case, that children are very soon after birth exposed without covering, both to the scorching heat of the sun and to the chilling dews of night. Not a single instance of trismus in infants, or even of tetanus in adults, occurred to my notice in Africa, neither have the natives any knowledge of the complaint. In the West Indies, negro children are very liable to locked jaw soon after birth, which very generally proves fatal. The cause of this complaint is not certainly known ; some assert that it is a consequence of the meconium being retained, and that it may always be prevented by evacuating the bowels soon after birth by a little castor oil. Others have ascribed it to improper treatment of the navel string ; others, again, have referred it to the wood smoke with which their small confined huts are filled at nights; but this practice is universal in Africa, where the disease itself is unknown*. It is most common between the fifth and fourteenth days after birth, and it has been supposed that one fourth of the negro children in the West Indies are cut off by it. Until children are able to walk, they are carried upon their mothers backs, having their legs stretched round her waist †; they are supported in this situation by a cloth which passes round their bodies, and is tied upon the mother's breast, which leaves only their arms at liberty. In this posture children are often carried for several hours, while the mother is engaged in her houshold affairs. They often fall asleep in this situation, hav-

---

* Dr. Chisholm attributes the trismus nascentium, which, he says, does not happen after the *ninth* day, to cold and impure air. His friend, Dr. Stewart of Grenada, having observed, "that the Negro midwives were not very nice in their choice of the instrument with which they cut the umbilical cord, he suspected that the rubiginous particles might produce such irritation as to cause the fatal disease in question. Having this in view, he directed the midwives to dress the part with a folded piece of soft linen, well soaked in spirit of turpentine, instead of the common way. They attended to his directions, and not a single infant has died on the estate since." From this diversity of opinion among authors, we have reason to suspect that the true cause of this malady is yet unknown. Bajon asserts, that in Cayenne it is found only upon the coast, at a small distance from the sea : at the distance of eight, ten, or twelve miles inland, it never occurs. He further adds, it is found more frequently among those who live upon small hills or eminences directly exposed to the sea air, than among those who live in marshy situations, or are sheltered by mountains or woods from the sea breeze.

† This may perhaps account for their legs being so frequently curved.

ing their naked heads exposed to a scorching sun, without experiencing any bad effects. Upon the Kroo Coast, children are carried behind their mothers backs in a kind of small basket. Sometimes they are placed upon a mat, or suffered to roll at liberty upon the ground. Deformed children are very rarely seen, but when this misfortune happens, it does not diminish the care and anxiety of the mother: such a monster is unknown in Africa as a mother who would destroy her child because it is deformed. This is reported to be done among the North American Indians, though Dr. Rush says, it is the severity of the Indian manners which destroys infants.

Negro children are very subject, for the first two or three months, to a papulous eruption very much resembling the RED GUM. Owing to the little care which is taken to prevent it, they are seldom free from the KRA-KRAS. When children are thought to be long in learning to speak, or when they ARTICULATE INDISTINCTLY, the leaves of a plant called fooruntum brakky are burnt, and the ashes, mixed with palm oil, are rubbed over the lower part of the face and neck.

In cases of TINEA CAPITIS, the head is washed with a pretty strong infusion of red pepper in water, or with the country soap, which is very acrid.

Children are sometimes affected with swellings of the lower extremities, somewhat resembling ANASARCA, which soon prove fatal if improperly treated. This complaint is called by the Soosoos kayberree, and by the Bulloms and Timmanees yefoó; it is cured by the repeated exhibition of emetics and active purgatives.

TUMEFIED GLANDS of the neck are called by the Soosoos bolay, by the Bulloms boómboo, and by the Timmanees opoff, but they do not apply of any particular treatment.

Children who appear puny, and do not THRIVE WELL, are washed with a variety of vegetable infusions, which are generally of an astringent nature, and used cold. Among others, the leaves of the cayaba, amaryllis ornata, are infused in cold water, and used every morning for a length of time; in like manner, the fresh leaves of koonto are bruised, and infused in cold water, to wash the child with every morning. Among the Kroo people, when a child is sickly, the leaves of ximenioides or monkey apple, which they call prang-fa, are infused in water, and when the child is washed with the decoction, the leaves are also rubbed over its body. The same people, when a child is long before it walks, use the following superstitious method : if a boy, they take four, if a girl, only three of the exuviæ or skins of spiders; these they burn, and mixing the ashes with a little palm oil, they rub it well on the inside of the wrists and ancles. In cases of DIARRHŒA, a weak infusion of the bark of the mangrove tree, rhizophora mangle, is made use of.

African children are very subject to prodigious large protrusions of the navel, or EXOMPHALOS, which are sometimes larger than a man's fist; this they look upon as a great deformity and wish to avoid. Atkins imagines it to be " the effect of bad midwifery, or straining in their infancy to walk." It more probably arises from relaxation of the parts, and from the want of a bandage round the child's body to support the umbilicus until it has acquired a sufficient degree of firmness. It is a very rare occurrence among the Nova Scotian settlers at Free Town, who use moderate pressure upon the part for some months after birth.

I have seen only one instance of RICKETS among them; this occurred in the child of a white man by a Mulatto woman, but which had been entirely brought up among the natives. The child was about eight years old when I saw her; she had recovered from the disease, but her joints were much enlarged, and the legs and arms were very crooked.

In cases of PROLAPSUS ANI, the bark of tansai, is boiled in water, and the decoction given internally; at the same time, the expressed juice of a plant, called by the Soosoos labba-labby, is applied frequently to the part affected.

I have never seen nor heard of an instance of hare-lip among them, but Atkins mentions a case which he saw himself. Herodotus informs us, that among some of the African Nomades, it was the custom, when the child had reached its fourth year, to cauterize the veins on the crown of the head, or temples, with new shorn wool, in order to dry up the pituita. To this mode of practice these people referred their good state of health. Herodotus adds, that the Africans enjoy better health than any other people, though he is uncertain whether it be from this cause. When convulsions are produced by the above practice, the same author observes, they are cured by sprinkling the children with goats' urine *. The actual cautery is not at present used by the Africans, neither does goats' urine make a part of their materia medica.

That strange propensity, called DIRT EATING in the West Indies, where it frequently occurs among the slaves, and often proves fatal by inducing chronic complaints, is sometimes met with among the children in Africa. When this pernicious practice has been followed for some time, it induces such a change in the countenance and complexion, as renders the disease at first sight obvious to every one. The colour of the skin changes from a deep black to a dirty light brown, or even approaches to a clay colour. The skin also feels rough, and is cold to the touch. The tunica conjunctiva, or white of the eye, becomes of a dusky yellowish white. The countenance appears dejected, the eye-lids are puffy, and the whole face is bloated. The gums lose their healthy red colour, becoming pale and flaccid, and the inside of the lips and tongue appear almost white ; even the hair undergoes a change of colour, and becomes of a dirty white, like that of the white negro. There is a

* Melpom. 187.

constant uneasy aching pain at the stomach, attended with a degree of nausea and loathing of food. The pulse at first is not much affected, but gradually becomes quicker, and very small; there is frequently a troublesome palpitation of the heart, and a constant throbbing of the large vessels in the lower part of the neck. The respiration is often oppressed, and is always hurried by the least degree of exercise. The abdominal viscera, particularly the mesenteric glands, being enlarged and hardened, cause the belly to swell; the lower extremities become anasarcous; and frequently towards the conclusion of the disease, effusion takes place into the cavities of the abdomen and thorax.

These unhappy people are fondest of a white kind of clay, resembling tobacco pipe clay, with which they fill their mouths, and allow it to dissolve gradually. In the West Indies there are persons who make it into cakes, and privately sell it to slaves having this depraved appetite*. Mr. Edwards in his remarks on the subject, says, " they become dropsical, and complain of a con-

* Upon dissection " the stomach is found much enlarged, and thickened in its coats; the liver sometimes enlarged and schirrous, but always preternaturally white; the gall bladder sometimes filled with biliary concretions; the bile never of a healthy appearance, generally thin and watery, and slightly yellow or green; the mesenteric glands indurated and schirrous."—In the cure " much benefit has been derived from weak fermented liquors—acescent cane-liquor has cured many."

" It is remarkable that negroes, subject to this disease, have been much benefited by living in a low situation, near marshes, which quickly prove fatal to whites." Medical and Physical Journal. vol. ii. 172.

stant uneasiness in the stomach; for which they find a temporary relief in eating some kind of earth. The French planters call this disease mal d'estomac*, or the stomach evil. The best and only remedy is, kind usage and wholesome animal food; and perhaps a steel drink may be of some service †." The natives of Africa endeavour to cure children of this morbid appetite by exciting in them a disgust towards such substances; they mix them therefore with pepper, or any kind of filth, and oblige the children to lick the mixture off the ground. Sometimes one of the large lizards, with a red head, called by the Bulloms tek, which is generally found upon trees, is dried, powdered, and mixed with the bark of a tree. Of this preparation the patient is obliged to take a dose every morning, mixed with water, until the whole be consumed.

Many children at certain times have prodigiously LARGE BELLIES, but I never saw any symptoms of disease attending this appearance. They do not attribute it to worms, nor is any attention paid to it, as it always disappears spontaneously.

---

* Anasarca Americana Sauvagesii.

† History of the West Indies.

APPENDIX. N° I.

AN

ACCOUNT OF CIRCUMCISION,

AS IT IS PRACTISED ON THE

WINDWARD COAST OF AFRICA.

HERODOTUS has been censured for asserting that the Egyptians were the first who used circumcision, and that other nations borrowed the practice from them *. But in this respect he does not merit blame, as he drew his

---

* The words of Herodotus are, " The Colchians, Egyptians, and Ethiopians, are the only people who have used circumcision from the earliest times. The Phenicians and Syrians in Palestine confess that they learnt this custom from the Egyptians ; but the Syrians, who inhabit the rivers Thermodon and Parthenius, and the Macrones, who border upon them, say they lately learned it from the Colchians. These are the only people who use circumcision, and it appears that they do it after the same manner as the Egyptians." Herodotus appears to be in doubt, whether the custom of circumcising originated with the Egyptians or Ethiopians, but is inclined to think that the latter nation borrowed it from the former one, because the Phenicians, who traded with the Greeks, discontinued the practice of circumcision in imitation of them. As Herodotus informs us that the Colchians sprung from the Egyptians, and were of a dark colour, and had crisp or curled hair, of course both these nations, as well as the Ethiopians, were real negroes, and, no doubt, received this practice from the same source.

information from the Egyptian priests, who, in order to establish the antiquity of their nation, laid claim to the origin of this custom. It is probable, however, that there was no such custom among the Egyptians even in the time of Moses: a negative is fairly deducible from the expression of the " reproach of Egypt" being taken away from the Israelites, when the practice of circumcision was revived in the wilderness by Joshua. At what period, subsequent to the time of Moses, it was adopted by the Egyptians, we are not informed: but we may conclude, that a custom of this kind would be readily received by a people so much addicted to superstition, and among whom every ceremony had some mystical meaning attached to it.

The practice of circumcision, considering the circumstances under which it was introduced, was likely to be rapidly extended. All the children of Abraham, it is to be presumed, were enjoined to follow his example; and the reverence which, in the patriarchal ages, was paid to the heads of families, would prevent any deviation from customs which they had introduced or sanctioned. The example of a man so greatly respected as Abraham must have had great weight also amongst his cotemporaries. Their minds must have been impressed by seeing an old man, at the advanced age of ninety-nine years, submit to so painful an operation, and cause it to be performed upon every male in his family: they would be impressed

by the religious solemnities which were probably
used on the occasion; and they might also be
influenced to adopt the practice by superstitious
motives. We have a proof in the melancholy
history of the people of Schechem, recorded in
the thirty-fourth chapter of Genesis, of the facility
with which, on much slighter grounds, this innova-
tion was received by the inhabitants of a large town.
This institution has been by some considered as
little better than a species of exorcism. Philo supposes it was performed, to guard against a disease
called anthrax, which, in the eastern countries, is
said to affect those parts when left in their natural
state. This anthrax was probably nothing more
than an excoriation, arising from acrid matter retained behind the glans, a circumstance which
occurs more rarely in warm climates, than is commonly supposed *. Some of the Africans assert, that
they use circumcision to prevent their contracting
the venereal disease. This idea may be thought
to be corroborated by an observation of Dr. Russel,

* In Professor Michaelis's " Questions proposées à une Societé
de Savants," is an observation respecting the utility of circumcision in obviating the effects of a natural phimosis, which, though
the complaint occur more rarely than is imagined, merits consideration. Mr. Niebuhr mentions an instance of a christian at
Mosul, where in all probability circumcision would have proved
serviceable. He is not of opinion that circumcision is necessary
to health in hot climates because " the Parsîs, or disciples of
Zoroaster, who are also called Guebres, or adorers of fire, the
Pagans of the Indies, and some Caffre nations in Africa, who all
live in climates as warm as the Mahometans of Arabia, do not circumcise, and yet enjoy as good health as the Jews, Mahometans.
and some Caffre nations who use circumcision."

who says, that "the Christians seemed more liable to slight venereal infection than the Turks, who seldom had a gonorrhœa unattended with more formidable symptoms." Another reason, according to Philo, for performing this operation, is to increase fecundity; and he asserts, that those nations who practise it are more fruitful than those who do not. The futility of this argument, however, is very evident, as we are certain that the prepuce can in no wise affect the act of procreation, unless by constriction it should oppose a mechanical obstacle.

Circumcision, though universally practised by the Mahometan nations, is not mentioned in the Koran. In the Sonna, which like the Mishna or second law of the Jews, is the oral law of the Mohammedans, and contains the sayings and actions of Mahomet, which are not related in the Koran, but which being first handed down by tradition, were afterwards committed to writing, it is said that circumcision is a necessary rite for men; and for women, honourable. "Circumcision," Dr. Russel says, "is termed by Mahomet *sonna*, which, according to the explanation of Reland, does not comprehend things absolutely necessary, but such as though the observance of them be meritorious; their neglect is not liable to punishment *." Among the Mahometan nations in Africa, this operation is generally performed about the age of of thirteen. In this they imitate the Arabians,

* History of Aleppo.

who, after the example of Ishmael, their reputed progenitor, have fixed that age for its performance.

Among the Bulloms and Timmanees, the ceremony takes place at any age, from the first month to the thirteenth or fourteenth year. The manner of performing it among the Bulloms, which I once witnessed, was as follows. Early in the morning the boys were assembled : after squatting down upon the hams, every one of them put a finger upon the edge of a large shallow brass dish, called a neptune, in which were placed an ear of Indian corn, a single kola, a piece of iron, and a sharp-pointed sword, as offerings to Griffee, the evil genius : at the same time the head man of the village, who presided at the ceremony, made a long prayer, that the boys might all speedily recover, and none of them die, which sometimes happens. When he had prayed, they were led into a cool shady grove, near the town. The operator, who was also a gree-gree-maker, dipping his forefinger* into some wood ashes, made a mark with it upon the prepuce, immediately over the corona glandis. He then laid hold of the prepuce with the forefinger and thumb of the left hand, and drawing it forwards as much as possible, with a common gardener's knife he cut or rather haggled through it at the place where he had made the mark. In this manner eight boys, from five years of age to about twelve or thirteen, were circumcised. The hemorrhage, which was

---

* The Mandingos use the thumb nail for this purpose.

H H

inconsiderable, was restrained by an infusion of the leaves of a plant called by the Bulloms, from a fancied resemblance, nwee tee kell, or monkey's ear. It grows close to the ground, and bears a red fruit not unlike a strawberry. Until the cure, which commonly requires two or three weeks, be completed, the boys pass their time while the sun is above the horizon in this shady place. After sunset they are permitted to leave their confinement and return to their own habitations, in which they may remain till near sunrise. In general no other application is made to the wound than the bark of the maylip, finely powdered, and sprinkled over it; sometimes a little ground chalk is used to absorb the moisture. In the Rio Nunez, the boys who undergo this operation are withdrawn from public view for the space of several weeks, during which time they are instructed in various religious ceremonies*.

---

* Among the Jews circumcision is still performed on the eighth day. The instrument used for the purpose is generally a knife of stone. The child being held by the father or godfather, the operator lays hold of the prepuce and cuts it off, after which he applies his mouth to the part, and sucks the blood, which he spits into a bowl of wine, and then sprinkles some styptic powder upon the wound. The operation is performed by no particular person or set of people, but the office of operator is considered by them as honourable. This is contrary to the opinion of the Arabians, who look upon the operation as indelicate, and therefore hold the operator in contempt. It is thus described by Niebuhr: " Dans cette operation on tire le prepuce qu'on serre avec une pincette, le barbier est quelquefois obligé de souffler avec la bouche dans l'orifice, & il arrive alors que le pauvre enfant de crainte de douleur, laisse echapper quelques gouttes de son eau."

Circumcision is also in use among the females upon some parts of the western coast of Africa, though much less generally than among the men. It is not practised by the women in the neighbourhood of Sierra Leone, and, indeed, is scarcely known to them. In the river Sherbró, however, which is inhabited by Bulloms, there is a society of girls called Sandee girls, who, besides being initiated into various mysteries, are instructed to dance in public. Before their admission into this order they are obliged to submit to the operation of circumcision, for which they give no other reason than that it is done to prevent those parts becoming too large by frequent motion. Circumcision prevails almost universally among the Foola, Mandingo, and Soosoo women. Several religious ceremonies accompany its performance. The girls are kept in a secluded place for two months, during which time they are not exposed to public view, except on very particular occasions, and even then their faces are concealed by a cloth. The ceremonies which usually accompany this practice, are thus described by a late amusing writer: " Every year during the dry season, and on the first appearance of a new moon, the girls of each town, who are judged marriageable, are collected together, and, in the night preceding the day on which the ceremony takes place, are conducted by the women of the village into the inmost recesses of a wood. Griggories or charms are placed at every avenue or path which might lead to the consecrated spot, to warn and deter the approach of the ignorant or designing, during their confinement, which continues one moon and one day. They are seen by no person but the old woman who performed the operation, and who brings them their provisions daily; should she, through sickness, or any other cause, be unable to attend, the person who is substituted in her place calls out with a loud voice as she approaches, leaves the victuals at a certain spot, and retires unseeing or unseen; for should any person, either through accident or design, break into their retirements, death is the punishment annexed.

It is principally during their confinement in the wood, when the body is subdued by pain, and the mind softened by the gloomy stillness of every thing around them, that they are taught the religious customs and superstitions of their country; for, till that period, they are not thought capable of understanding or practising them.—When the time destined for their continuance in the wood is expired, which is judged sufficient for the healing of their wounds, they are brought into the town in the night, where they are received by all the women of the village, young and old, quite naked: in this state, and in a kind of irregular procession, with various instruments of national music, they parade the streets till break of day, and should any man be found even peeping during their peregrination, he would immediately suffer death, or pay a slave.—A probation of one moon succeeds their release from the wood, during which they are every day conducted in procession, with music, and their heads and bodies covered, to every principal person's house in the town, before which they dance and sing till they are presented with some trifling present. At the expiration of the month they are released from further attendance, and immediately given to the men destined for their husbands*, who give a public entertainment upon the occasion."

The cool of the morning is the time chosen for the performance of the operation, which is done by an old woman, whose peculiar province it is. At Teembo, in the Foola country, they are very strict in enforcing this custom, but in the more remote parts of the kingdom they are much less so ; and it is even said, in some instances, to be neglected until the person be grown old. For what reason it is performed at an advanced age, or whether it be merely to avoid the obloquy which in these countries attaches to those who have not undergone this operation is uncertain. There is reason to believe it is not practised by any nation to the northward of Sierra Leone, except by those who profess Mahommedanism †. It is difficult to

---

* Matthew's Voyage to Sierra Leone.

† Among the inhabitants of Bambouc it is the custom to circumcise their children, both male and female. This is done, says a French writer, " to give them liberty to marry ; for it would be a great crime for a young man or woman to give themselves up to debauchery before they were circumcised : thus circumcision appears to give them liberty to abandon themselves to pleasure, without remorse, and without incurring the smallest censure. This ceremony is performed once every year : they begin with the boys. Every where else it is a marabou who performs the operation ; but as the natives of Bambouc are wise enough to have

say how far this custom extends to the south of
Sierra Leone. Dr. Issert asserts, that it is not
the custom among the women at Akra, though
universally practised by the men. In the kingdom of Dahomy, Mr. Dalzel informs us, that " a
certain operation, peculiar to this country, is likewise performed upon the women ;" and in a note
he adds, " Prolongatio, videlicet, artificialis labio-
rum pudendi, capellæ mamillis simillima." This

no marabous, the honour of exercising the priesthood belongs to
the master of the village.

" The ceremony begins with the noise of drums and other instruments. The master of the village kills a bullock, which he buys
for the occasion, and all the company partake of it. When the
repast is finished, the people make a kind of procession : the
musicians walk first, the girls and boys follow, walking two and
two ; after them come all the inhabitants of the village, making
terrible cries. When they have arrived at the place where the
operation is to be performed, they divide into two bands, the
boys on one side, and the girls on the other. The head of the
village then comes forward with a knife in his hand, which he
makes use of to remove the prepuces ; these are carefully pre-
served, and put into a vessel, which the chief buries with great
respect. He makes also an incision upon the girls, and buries
apart the small portion of which he deprives them.

" After this ceremony, the circumcised have a right to go and
seek their victuals any where but at home, during the space of
forty days, in which time they wander about the country, without being permitted to have any communication with the girls,
who wander about in like manner. In order to prevent any
communication, some of the mamayambaus, whom the natives
look upon as sorcerers, rub their bodies with a kind of clay,
cover themselves with branches of trees, and run with a whip in
their hand after the young girls and boys. When they meet
them, they execute their office very rudely, to the great satisfaction of the fathers and mothers, who make a point of feasting
the mamayambaus well during the whole of the time prescribed
to their children to observe continence." Voyage au Pays de
Bambouc.

operation does not appear to resemble circumcision, but probably is analogous to a custom among the Hottentot females, of stretching the nymphæ by weights appended to them, or by some other means, to an enormous length, which Linnæus has distinguished by the term " sinus pudoris*." Among the Mahommedan nations on this part of the coast, the operation consists in removing the nymphæ, together with the præ-putium clitoridis, not the clitoris itself, as has been imagined ; this is corroborated by Dr. Schotte, who appears to have examined the subject with great accuracy. In a letter to Professor Stein, speaking of the females of Senegal, among whom the practice of circumcision is observed, he says, " les Mauresses, non pas les Negresses sont toutes cir-concises d'une façon, ayant les nymphes & les clitoris coupés pour diminuer les parties molles : j'en ai examiné plusieurs en vie, & je n'ai trouvé le moindre vestige si non que des petites cicatrices, & il y en avoit, qui se souviennent de l'operation etant enfans †." Mr. Bruce appears to entertain nearly the same ideas upon this subject : he ob-

---

* Owing to this cause the Hottentots have rather too hastily been supposed to have some peculiarity in those parts. Buffon says, they have " une espece d'excroissance ou de peau dure & large qui leur croit au dessus de l'os pubis, & qui descend jusqu'au milieu des cuisses en forme de tablier," (Hist. Nat. de l'Homme) ; but Dr. Sparrman positively asserts, " that the women have no parts uncommon to the rest of their sex."

† Sommering ueber die korperliche verschiedenheit des ne-gers, &c.

serves, that the practice of circumcision, or, as he
calls it, excision, is universally followed among the
women in Abyssinia and other neighbouring nations. " All the Egyptians," he says, " the Arabians, and nations to the south of Africa, the
Abyssinians, Gallas, Agows, Gafats, and Gongas,
make their children undergo this operation, at no
fixed time indeed, but always before they are marriageable *." The same author refers the origin of
this custom to a certain mal-conformation or redundancy of parts among the women of those
countries. " From climate or some other cause," he
continues, " a certain disproportion is found generally to prevail among them," and, " they endeavour to remedy this deformity by the amputation
of that redundancy." In opposition to this opinion,
it may be very confidently affirmed, that whatever
reason the females on the western coast of Africa,
who follow this practice, may have for continuing
it, and it is doubtful if there be any but custom
immemorially established, there is at least no phy-

---

* A recent traveller, speaking of the practice of excision, says,
" it consists in *cutting off the clitoris* a little before the period of
puberty, or at about the age of eight or nine years." Thirteen
or fourteen young females underwent this operation in a house
where he was. " It was performed by a woman ; and some of
them complained much of the pain, both at and after it. They
were prevented from locomotion, but permitted to eat meat. The
parts were washed every twelve hours with warm water, which
profuse suppuration rendered necessary. At the end of eight
days the greater part were in a condition to walk, and liberated
from their confinement. Three or four of them remained under
restraint till the thirteenth day." Browne's Travels in Africa.

sical cause for it. Moreover, the redundancy or mal-conformation of parts above mentioned, is more rarely met with in these countries than in Europe; and where the custom of circumcision is unknown, which is probably over the greater part of the continent, no complaint is made on this head. We are informed by Dr. Russel, that the circumcision of females is not known at Aleppo. It is termed there *bitre*; and he adds, " consistit in incisione nymphæ puellaris."

Mr. Niebuhr says, this operation is performed on most of the females of Oman, at least in the country of Sohar; it is practised also by most of those who inhabit both sides of the Persian gulf and Basra, as well as by the Mahommedan women and Copts in Egypt, and by those of Habbesch, and of Cambay, near Surat. At Bagdad, the Arab women circumcise their daughters. The Turkish women do not follow this custom, and as we depart from the frontiers of Arabia, fewer women are found circumcised in the Turkish towns*. Speaking of the utility of the practice, Niebuhr says, " apparemment que les femmes en retirent l'avantage de se laver avec plus de facilitè. Un marchand Arabe m'en donna cependant encore une autre raison, savoir, qu'on veut par là empecher l'erection du clitoris, nommé sünbula en Arabe : & cet homme pensoit, que la decence l'exigeoit."

---

* Mr. Forskal learnt that the circumcision of girls was customary at Mokha, but not at Sana, nor among the Arab Jews.

Mr. Niebuhr further adds, " that the women who circumcise the girls at Kahira are as publicly known there as midwives are in Europe; and when they are wanted they are called out of the street, a proof that no great ceremony attends it. The time for performing this operation is the tenth year."

APPENDIX. Nº II.

AFRICAN BARK.

THE BELLENDA* is a tree of considerable mag‑
nitude, though I do not recollect to have seen
it growing; neither do I know of what nature its
wood is, nor to what œconomical purposes it is
applied by the natives. The bark that was sent
to me, consisted of pieces as large as the hand,
and full half an inch in thickness. On the outside
it was very scabrous and unequal, full of deep fis‑
sures, and covered with large patches of a grey‑
coloured lichen. The inner surface was of a deeper
red, and smoother than the external, but had some‑
what of a granulated appearance. It was very fri‑
able, and when broken in a longitudinal direction,
exhibited a number of pale small fibres, disposed
in strata, and inclosed in a substance of a darker

---

* This is ranked above, page 45, as a species of Rondeletia, but
perhaps incorrectly. Mr. Afzelius had been informed that the
bark used at the Rio Nunez was obtained from a tree similar to
one which grows in Sierra Leone, and which he found to be a
Rondeletia. In consequence of this information he brought to
London a considerable quantity of the bark from Sierra Leone;
but, upon examination and trials, it differed both in taste, colour,
and chemical properties, from the Rio Nunez bark, nor was it,
when given medicinally, attended with the same beneficial
effects.

red colour. These fibres appeared more evidently when the bark was broken transversely, for then a number of whitish points were seen, which in a strong light had a shining or silvery appearance, being, as it were, set in the red coloured substance. When chewed, the bark felt gritty to the tongue, tinged the saliva with a slight red colour, and imparted a considerable degree of astringency, not unpleasant to the taste, but unaccompanied with the slightest bitterness.

This bark is nearly devoid of smell, and possesses scarcely any aroma: it is of a very fixed nature, and does not easily impart its virtues to water. One drachm of it finely powdered was triturated for ten minutes in three ounces of pure water, and afterwards passed through filtering paper. The filtered liquid did not appear to have taken up much of the colouring principle; and an ounce measure of it, very accurately weighed, was found to have acquired only two grains of additional weight. To half an ounce of the above infusion, five drops of a filtered solution of sal martis, containing a scruple of the salt dissolved in one ounce of water, were added: the fluid immediately changed to a dark blue colour, but still retained a degree of transparency; at the end of three days it turned to a dirty blackish green, but deposited no sediment.

An ounce of the bark in fine powder was infused for four hours in a pint of water, in a heat of 150°, but during the last ten minutes in a boiling

heat. The liquor when filtered appeared of a
dusky brown colour; and an ounce measure of it
was found to have acquired three grains more than
the same quantity of pure water. Five drops of
the martial solution, added to half an ounce of
the above infusion, immediately changed it to a
deep brown, and afterwards to a dirty blue colour.

An ounce of the bark, rather coarsely powdered,
was boiled for an hour, in twenty-four ounces of
pure water, and filtered while hot. This decoction
had acquired a dark red colour, and was beautifully transparent when held up to the light. An
ounce of it had gained five grains of additional
weight. To half an ounce of this decoction were
added five drops of the martial solution, when it
immediately assumed a deep black colour: at the
end of three days it deposited a dark coloured
sediment, much more abundant than in any of the
former infusions; whilst the clear fluid above remained of a dark green colour.

Half an ounce of the bark in fine powder was infused for twenty-four hours in a pint of cold water,
and several times agitated: when filtered, the
liquor had only acquired a slight duskiness of colour, and very much resembled the infusion made
by trituration with cold water. To half an ounce
of this infusion five drops of martial solution were
added; the mixture did not lose its transparency,
but assumed rather a darker colour; and at the
end of two days deposited a small quantity of a
light brownish fæcula. One drachm of the fine
powder, triturated with half a drachm of mild

magnesia, in three ounces of water, for ten minutes, and afterwards filtered, was found to have gained three grains and a quarter of additional weight in each ounce. The filtered infusion appeared of a transparent orange colour, which by the addition of the martial solution acquired immediately a dirty black, void of transparency; at the end of three days a dark coloured sediment was deposited, the superincumbent fluid remaining of a dusky brown. Half an ounce of spirit of wine, added to an equal quantity of the decoction of this bark, produced no other change than to render the colour a little paler; at the end of a few hours, however, a flocculent sediment was deposited. One drachm of the fine powder, triturated for ten minutes with half a drachm of mild kali, in three ounces of water, was found, when filtered, to have acquired only one grain in each ounce: the liquor was of a very deep red, but had scarcely any other taste than that of an alcali.

Tinctures were made from the bark, by infusing two drachms of coarse powder, for ten days, in an ounce and half of proof spirit : this was repeated with the same quantity of spirit of wine, sweet spirit of vitriol, and sweet spirit of nitre. An ounce of the filtered tincture, made with proof spirit, had taken up three grains; that with spirit of wine, three grains and a quarter; that with sweet spirit of vitriol, four grains; and that with sweet spirit of nitre, which exhibited the deepest colour, had gained seven grains.

The only opportunity I had of using this bark

in Africa was in cases of diarrhœa, where opiates and astringents were indicated: it was generally used by me at that time in decoction, in which form it proved very effectual, and was sufficiently grateful to the stomach to render its exhibition easy. The three following cases, which occurred soon after my return to England, afford some proof of its febrifuge power.

Jan. 7, 1797, Mr. T. about thirty-three years of age, of rather a fair complexion and full habit of body, was suddenly seized, on the 4th inst. after exposure to cold, with a severe pain over the left orbit of the eye, extending over the side of the head. The pain is ushered in by a febrile paroxysm, preceded by slight chillness, and returns every succeeding day at eleven A. M. continuing with unabated violence until three P. M. when a partial sweat breaks out about the neck and breast, which terminates the attack. This day he was obliged to walk a mile from home just before the paroxysm was expected, which has greatly aggravated it. He is ordered to go to bed immediately, and to take tinct. opii, g^{tt} xxv; and when the paroxysm has subsided, to take a drachm of cort. African. every two hours.—Jan. 8, noon. He did not feel the slightest relief yesterday from the opiate, the pain continued severe until evening, and after its subsidence he was obliged to walk home. During the night he took nearly an ounce of the powdered bark. The paroxysm returned this morning sooner than usual, and is at present extremely severe. He now is to omit the bark, and not to resume its use until the accession be finished. He is desired to take the opiate to-morrow, two hours before the return of the fit is expected, and to continue in bed.—Jan. 9, noon. The exacerbation of yesterday was extremely severe, and continued with unabating violence until five P. M. when it gradually subsided. He has taken an ounce and half of the bark since yesterday evening, and feels at present only a slight pain over one eye. The bark is to be continued. There has been no return of the fit yesterday nor to-day. The remedy was continued a day or two longer, during which time the patient exposed himself to the open air as usual, and has suffered no relapse.

Jan. 19, 1797. Mrs. A. aged forty, of a brown complexion, has been for a week past affected every morning, between seven and eight o'clock, with a severe cold fit of ague, followed by increased heat, and terminating about five P. M. in a profuse perspiration. She took an emetic last night, which operated well, and was ordered to take an anodyne draught this morning about two hours before the expected return of the paroxysm. Notwithstanding the opiate, the fit returned to-day at the usual time, with no alteration in the symptoms. She is ordered to begin at six in the evening to take two scruples of the African bark, and to repeat it every hour until the time of the next paroxysm.—Jan. 20, noon. She has taken during the night an ounce of the bark, but without preventing the return of the paroxysm: the cold fit has, however, been much less severe, and of shorter duration than before. The head-ache was very acute, the pain being chiefly fixed over one eye; but it was relieved by an opiate, which excited a copious perspiration She is now ordered to take one drachm of the bark every hour, and an opiate two hours before the expected exacerbation.

Jan. 21, noon. Since last report, eleven doses of bark have been taken, which have agreed perfectly well with her stomach, and there has been no return of the paroxysm.—April 1, continues perfectly well.

Oct. 1, 1796, Mr. B. a sailor, aged forty, of a dark complexion and robust habit, for a week past has been affected every day, about nine in the morning, with a most excruciating pain on the left side of the head and face, but felt most severely over the left orbit. This pain continues until four in the afternoon, when it is relieved by a partial sweat. He has experienced temporary relief from an opiate taken before the accession of the fit, when he at the same time confined himself to bed; but on exposing himself to the external air, the pain immediately returns with its usual violence. He had no anodyne yesterday, and underwent a very violent paroxysm; he is ordered to take ʒss. of the African bark every two hours, beginning at six P. M.

Oct. 2, noon. He has taken ʒi. of the bark, without any return of the fit, though he had no opiate, and walked all the morning in the open air. He repeated the bark two or three days longer, and continued free from complaint.

With the following case I was favoured by the late Dr. Cappe, of York, while he officiated as assistant physician to the Public Dispensary in London.

June 8, 1798. Nicholas White, aged 54, an Irishman, has been a gentleman's servant for the greater part of his life.

About thirty years ago he had an intermittent fever, in Ireland, the paroxysms of which returned regularly every evening for about a week. He then employed charms, and the disease left him for a week, but returned again at the end of a fortnight from the first attack; but the type of the fever was changed, the paroxysm returning only every other day, sometimes at noon, sometimes about seven o'clock in the evening. When he had been ill about five months, he took half a pint of brandy, in which an ounce of tobacco had been infused for twenty-four hours. This draught made him excessively sick, but the fever continued for three months after, without any abatement. The paroxysms at length, though not less frequent, grew less and less severe for about a fortnight, and the fever left him entirely in the month of October, though he had used no other remedies of any kind.

Four years ago he entered the corps of artillery, as a driver of the field pieces. He was on the continent in French Flanders, about two years, and enjoyed perfectly good health while abroad. On his return to England, in Christmas 1795, he was employed as a labourer in the king's works at Purfleet.

On the 27th of July, 1796, about two o'clock P. M. while he was at work, he was seized with a paroxysm of fever. The fever returned daily for a fortnight, being every day a little later. The third fit happened about four P. M. The fever had continued about fortnight, when the period changed, and the paroxysms returned only every other day : they happened at later and later hours, till at length they came on at midnight, and afterwards early in the morning. In March, 1797, the fever assumed the quartan type. For the three last months a paroxysm has happened regularly every fourth day at seven P. M. The whole duration of the paroxysm is now about five hours. When the fever first assumed the quartan period, the cold fit lasted about two hours and a half, the hot and sweating stage together, about three hours and a half.

He continued to work at Purfleet till October, in the year 1796 ; he then came to London : but in November he left London and went into Essex, where he was employed in very easy service in the house of a gentleman, in whose family he had formerly been a servant. While he was in Essex he took bark, about two tea spoonfuls, in red wine, three times a day, but it had no effect on his fever : he employed charms too with as little success. In May, 1797, he returned to London, and has since that time taken no medicines. He is now employed in standing, at night, in Norfolk-street, Strand, with advertisements of the exhibition of Androides: but on the nights of the fever he is obliged to stay at home.

He believes that none of the other labourers at Purfleet had intermittents at the time he was seized with the fever.

He never observed whether the paroxysms, when they returned every day, were alternately more and less severe.

His countenance is now very sallow, his tongue furred, white on the edges, but yellowish in the middle.

Jan. 8. He expects the return of his fever to-morrow evening, Jan. 9.

Capiat pulv. ipec. gr. xv. vespere et cras mane calom. gr. iii.

Jan. 10. The emetic operated, but the calo-mel did not. His tongue is white but clean. He had a cold fit last night, less severe than usual: it lasted about an hour and a half; and was followed by a hot fit, which, with the sweating stage, lasted about two hours and a half, being also much less severe than usual.

Capiat cort. Africanæ ʒiss quotidie.

Jan. 15. On Friday the 12th he had no cold fit; but he had the hot fit at half past eight P. M. it lasted half an hour; he sweated also about half an hour. He looks better. Repetatur cortex.

Jan. 19. He had no fit on Monday 15th, nor on Thursday 18th. Repr.

Jan. 22. He had no fit on Sunday 21st.

Capiat cort. ʒi quotidie.

Jan. 27. He had no fit on the 24th. His complexion has gradually improved, and is now nearly natural.

℞ Cort. cascarill. contus. ʒii.
Aq font. ℔iii. coque ad ℔ii. Adde
Tinct. Cascarill. ʒiv.
M. capiat cochl. ii. vel iii. bis terve quotidie.——

Feb. 7. He has continued to take the corroborant mixture. He has had no return of fever, nor any uneasy symptoms. Since the 15th of last month he has exposed himself every night to the weather at his post in Norfolk-street.

Doctor Clark has exhibited the African bark in the infirmary at Newcastle with complete success in several cases of intermittents, and coincides with Doctor Willan and Dr. Cappe in thinking it a valuable accession to the materia medica. The high price of Peruvian bark, the uncertainty of obtaining a constant and regular supply of it during the time of war, and the schemes of interested men to enhance its value and lower its quality, render it an object of importance for us to increase the number of substitutes. The BELLENDA appears worthy of being ranked in that class : though the cases adduced in its favour are too few for any strong inferences to be drawn, yet, the recommendation of physicians eminent in their profession, and possessing such a share of public esteem, must excite others to make further trials with this bark, when a sufficient quantity of it is imported

APPENDIX. N° III.

SINCE writing the above, I have perused Mr. White's work on the regular gradation in man, in which, as far as regards the African, he adopts nearly the same sentiments with Professor Soemmering; but as some of the arguments adduced by Mr. White to establish his hypothesis, appear to rest upon too slight, and others upon a false foundation, and as the character of this writer may procure for them a reception to which they are not entitled, I think it right to subjoin a few observations, which a residence of near four years in Africa has enabled me to make.

As the chief deviations in the skeleton of the African from that of the European occur in the bony structure of the skull, and as these are given more concisely by Mr. White than by Professor Soemmering, they are here inserted from the work of the former. " I next examined the skull, and found the frontal and occipital bones narrower in the negro than in the European; the *foramen mag-num* of the occipital bone situated more backward, and the occipital bone itself pointing upwards, and forming a more obtuse angle with the spine in the former, than in the latter. The internal capacity of the skull was less in the former; and the fore parts of the upper and lower jaw, where they meet, were considerably more prominent. In the negro, the depth of the lower jaw, betwixt the teeth and the chin, was less; and that of the upper, betwixt the nose and the teeth, was greater: the distance from the back part of the *occiput* to the *meatus auditorius* was less, and from thence to the fore teeth was greater. The fore teeth were larger, not placed so perpendicularly in their sockets, and projecting more at their points than in Europeans: the angle of the lower jaw was nearer to a right angle, and the whole apparatus for mastication was stronger. The bones of the nose projected less. The chin, instead of projecting, receded. The *meatus auditorius* was wider. The bony sockets, which contained the eyes, were more capacious. The bones of the leg and thigh more gibbous: and, by the marks which were left upon the skull, it plainly appeared that the temporal muscles had been much larger. In all these points it differed from the European, and approached to the ape."

Having had no opportunity of examining the skeleton of a negro, I am unable to offer any remarks upon the above observations. But admitting their accuracy, it may be objected, that the result of a few comparative examinations ought not to be assumed as a standard; particularly as we frequently witness the occurrence of great and striking varieties in the bony compages even of Europeans. Mr. White points out the chin of the negro as deserving peculiar attention; this is also noticed by Professor Blumenbach (mentum retractius *.) This receding of the chin appears to be merely relative, and occurs perhaps only where the lips are remarkably protuberant †. We observe a great variety in this respect among Europeans. In some the lower incisors project beyond the upper ones, which renders the chin more prominent; in others, the chin recedes, which gives to the face a remarkable appearance of folly or simplicity.

An observation of Mr. White's, on which he insists strongly, appears not to have been noticed by any other writer, viz. that the arm, particularly the fore arm, is longer in the negro than in the European; a peculiarity which did not strike me in the living subject. Such varieties occur in England, but we are more apt to notice a remarkably short arm than a long one.

Professor Soemmering remarks, that the hands and feet of Negroes, are more flat than those of

* De Generis humani Varietate.

† This brings to my recollection a solitary instance of the receding chin in a black woman, who served as nurse to the hospital at Free Town, and who was called by a facetious friend of mine, " mother ·no chin." As a further proof that this is not a common occurrence, the Bulloms use it as a nickname, and say that such a person has " toot kin eeting, i. e. a (short) chin like a baboon.

Europeans, and their fingers and toes longer and smaller, a circumstance noticed by Mr. White; and that the knees are more distant from each other, or bowed, and the feet bent outwards. The only peculiarities which struck me in the black hand and foot were, the largeness of the latter, the thinness of the hand, and the flexibility of the fingers and toes. With their toes they can grasp a small stick, or even a piece of cord lying upon the ground. It is related of the American Indians, that they can distinguish persons of different nations by the print of the foot. It is easy to distinguish the impression of an African foot from that of an European, by the great divergency of the toes in the former; but the following pretence to acute discrimination in the natives of Zavilah, a town in Africa, cannot be admitted without a considerable degree of *credulity*: " Its inhabitants boast that they can distinguish people by the print of their feet, and can discover whether it be a stranger or an inhabitant, a man or a woman, a *robber* or a *slave*." Edrisius Hartmanni, p. 304.

The hands and feet are smaller, and more delicately formed, in the Sambo and Mulatto, than in the African, (or *genuine* Negro.)

Mr. White says, " Negroes sweat much less than Europeans; a drop of sweat being scarcely ever seen upon them." " Simiæ sweat still less, and dogs not at all." Here appears to be some proof of gradation, but the observation is altogether unfounded. When the African works in a hot sun, rivulets of sweat pour down his body. There is the same free discharge of insensible perspiration in him as in the European, causing his skin to be always cool and moist. The same variety indeed occurs in this respect among black people as among whites. Some perspire so readily, that on the least exertion the drops of sweat appear upon the skin like small pearls ; and it is with a view to restrain the tendency to profuse perspiration, that the practice of anointing with oil is so general in Africa.

With regard to the catamenia, Mr. White observes, " it is the general opinion of physiologists that females menstruate in larger quantities in warm climates than in cold ;"—" This may be true in Europeans, and in Creoles born of European parents, but I believe it is much otherwise in Negresses."—" Dr. Spaarman informs us, that those periods are much less troublesome to the female sex in Africa than in Europe." This last observation is just, but it is equally applicable to robust healthy women in England, and especially to such as use much exercise in the open air. I am unable to speak with more precision respecting this excretion in the natives of Africa, but among the settlers at Free Town, my opportunities of observation were very extensive. It may be proper to remark, that these people, who are generally called Nova Scotians, because brought from that country to Sierra Leone, are blacks, who were either carried to America when very young, or were born there of parents who came from Africa. Of course they are sufficiently acquainted with the customs of the white people, and they live nearly in the same way as the lower classes of people in Europe. Among the Nova Scotian women the catamenia have precisely the same appearance as in Europeans, who are equally exposed to the open air; and the same varieties occur with regard to quantity, periods of recurrence, &c. nor have they experienced any material alteration by change of climate. Mr. White, in consistency with the general law of gradation, for which he contends, observes, that " apes and baboons menstruate less than Negressés, monkies still less, and sapajous and sagouins not at all." It has been observed that bitches, and some other animals when in *heat*, have a discharge from the vagina ; of this kind probably is the discharge said to take place in some species of ape. Mr. White has not had ocular demonstration of the occurrence of this phenomenon in apes, though he has adduced, in support of it, the opinion of some eminent men : these, however, appear to have been gratuitously adopted, and may therefore be referred to the class of vulgar errors. The opinion is contradicted by an author of great reputation, who made the circumstance in question a particular object of enquiry for a number of years, and who explains the origin of the prevailing sentiment. Feminis contra non minus proprius sed magis universus & omnibus communis videtur *fluxus menstruus*, ita ut recte Plinium mulierem solum animal menstruale vocasse putem. Novi quidem aliis quoque animantibus femineis et quidem max-

ime ex quadrumanorum ordine, passim ab auctori-
bus tributum esse ejusmodi fluxum, simiam, v. c.
dianam ex caudæ apice menstruare dictum esse,
&c. At enim vero quoties a viginti inde annis
aut in vivariis aut a circumforaneis monstratas
femineas simias, papiones &c. mihi videre licuit,
de ea re quæsivi, et passim quidem unam alte-
ramve earum quandoque uterinæ hæmorrhagiæ
obnoxiam esse didici, quam vero in nulla peri-
odum servare, asserebant cordatiores custodes qui
ipsi eam pro morbosa contra naturæ ordinem affectione habe bant, quorumque plures candide fate-
bantur, vulgo eandem pro fluxu menstruo declarari
ut plebis admiratio eo major moveatur."

In speaking of the effects of climate, Dr. Spaarman, as quoted by Mr. White, observes, that
the Africans " never shewed the least signs of
being displeased with the hottest days of summer."
It is not surprising that the temperature of any
climate should be more congenial to the natives
than to foreigners; we see instances of this in the
southern and northern parts of Europe. Although Africans can support labour in the hottest
days with the same impunity as reapers in England in the dog days, yet they seek the shade in
preference, and are fond of plunging into water in
order to moderate the heat. Upon this subject
Mr. White further remarks, " West India planters
have assured me, and all writers agree, that the
Negroes in the West Indies suffer more from the
cold and moist weather, than from the warm and
dry ;" but this is also almost uniformly the case

with Europeans, who have resided for a considerable time in tropical climates. It is unnecessary
to observe, that cold and moisture have invariably
been found prejudicial to the human constitution;
and armies have always suffered much in the field
from this cause. The fatal effects of a warm state
of the air, when combined with moisture, have
been experienced too often by Europeans in hot
climates. Even the greatest degrees of natural
heat hitherto felt, when accompanied with a dry
state of the atmosphere, produce scarcely any other
effect upon Europeans than that of increasing
the irritability of the body; nor has any climate
been yet discovered too hot for their constitution.
A friend of mine, who resided some years in New
South Wales, assured me, that at a time when the
thermometer of Fahrenheit stood at 112° in the
shade, he was able to use exercise in the sun without much inconvenience, though the parroquets
dropped down dead from the excessive heat.

Mr. White continues, " when the blacks are
transported into these colder climates, they seem
to suffer more than we do from cold. I myself
have known instances where Negroes have lost
their toes by the frost, in circumstances wherein an
European would not have suffered. Consistently
with this, we find that the whole genus of simia is
impatient of cold; and no orang-outang has ever
yet been able to bear the cold of many European
winters."—We find a very great difference in
Europeans with respect to their capability of resisting the effects of cold; and such of them as

have resided long in tropical climates, manifest, on
their return to more northern regions, at least an
equal degree of susceptibility of cold with blacks.
From what I have seen in Africa, it would appear,
that the alternation of heat and cold is more indifferent to the African than is commonly supposed,
as he will sometimes sleep the whole night exposed to the open air, with the slightest covering,
though drenched with the copious and chilling dews
which fall in that country; while, at other times,
he sleeps in a close hut, heated by a large fire,
and filled with smoke. The fugitive blacks, who
joined the standard of the British army in America, supported the cold with as little inconvenience as the European soldiers. Many of them are
still resident in Nova Scotia, and appear to en-
dure the severity of winter as well as the whites.
Upwards of twenty African youths, from Sierra
Leone, were brought over to this country for education in 1799, and were placed in the neighbourhood of London, where many of them now are.
It does not appear by any means that they have
suffered more from the cold of winter, than European youths generally do.

On the duration of life, Mr. White observes,
" Negroes are shorter lived than Europeans. All
observations confirm the fact, that the children of
Negroes are more early and forward in walking
than those of Europeans; likewise that they arrive
at maturity sooner. The males are often ripe for
marriage at ten, and the females at eight years of
age." He observes, Negroes and Hottentots of

fifty are reckoned very old men. " In this respect, therefore, gradation is apparent ; for according to Linnæus, the orang-outang lives only twenty-five years." Whether Negroes be actually more short-lived than Europeans, and in that case, whether intemperance or the rigours of servitude may not be the cause, is uncertain. Among Europeans, it has been remarked, that sailors become sooner old and infirm than any other set of men ; and slaves, who are still more exposed to hardships, may become prematurely old from the same cause. The period of puberty is fixed in both sexes much too early. As far as my own experience goes, there is little difference in this respect between the African and the European. That their children walk early may be attributed to their being permitted to roll about upon the ground unincumbered with clothes.

With regard to the sexual parts, the law of gradation is certainly broken. Camper says, in the orang-outang, they resemble those of a dog ; the same author likewise asserts, that the knee of the orang is bent, and unfit for the erect posture. Tyson says, the orang wants the depending scrotum. Mr. White speaks of the scrotum being smaller in the Negro than European, but this escaped my notice ; and in twelve Negroes which he examined, four had no frænum præputii, " six of them had very trifling ones, which hardly could be called bridles; the remaining two were as perfect as Europeans."

It has already been asserted, that the circumcision of females is not practised on account of any disproportion in those parts. In Europe we frequently find elongations of the nymphæ, especially after child bearing.

The pendulous breasts of the African females have long been noticed by authors, but they are far from being general. I never saw an instance where women could " suckle their children upon their backs, by throwing the breasts over their shoulders ;" and it may be affirmed, that such a circumstance would occasion as much astonishment on the western coast of Africa as it would in Europe. A practice prevails of binding the breasts with a light bandage when turgid with milk, which must conduce to render them flabby. Even in England, however, the breasts grow to an immense size in persons who are disposed to become fat ; and among the lower classes of people, owing to the pernicious practice of suckling children for a great length of time, and to bad nourishment, as many instances of pendulous breasts are to be met with as in Africa, although the mode of dress prevents our noticing it.

THE MENTAL FACULTIES of the African next pass under the review of Mr. White, who has quoted, in confirmation of the theory of gradation, some passages from Mr. Jefferson's Notes on the State of Virginia. As the same quotations occur in Mr. Imlay's " Description of the Western Territory of North America," and are there accompanied by a complete refutation, I here insert them from that work.

Speaking of the Negroes, Mr. Jefferson says: " Comparing them by their faculties of memory, reason, and imagination, it appears to me, that in memory they are equal to the whites, in reason much inferior, as I think one could scarcely be found capable of tracing and comprehending the investigations of Euclid ; and that in imagination they are dull, tasteless, and anomalous. It would be unfair to follow them to Africa for this investigation ; we will consider them here* on the same stage of the whites, and where the facts are not apocryphal, on which a judgment is to be formed." " Can any position," says Mr. Imlay, " be more puerile and inconsistent ? ' We will consider them on the same stage of the whites, and then a comparison is not apocryphal.' Now I beg to know what can be more uncertain and false than estimating or comparing the intellect or talents of two descriptions of men ; one *enslaved, degraded, and fettered in all their acts of volition, without a vista through which the rays of light and science could be shot to illumine their ignorant minds*—the other free, independent, and with the advantage of appropriating the reason and science which have been the result of the study and labours of the philosophers and sensible men for centuries back ? If there have been some solitary instances where Negroes have had the advantages of education, they have shewn that they are in no degree inferior to whites, though they have always had in this

* In America.

country the very great disadvantage of associating only with their ignorant countrymen, which not only prevents that polish so essential to arrest admiration, but which imperceptibly leads to servility from the prevalence of manners."

" Mr. Jefferson's own arguments invalidate themselves." " Homer told us," he says, " nearly three thousand years since,

> " Jove fix'd it certain, that whatever day
> Makes man a slave, takes half his worth away."

" Now it is most certain, that the Negroes in America have not only been enslaved, but that they have existed under the most inhuman and nefarious tyranny, particularly in the southern states."

The following additional observations of Mr. Jefferson on this subject are taken from Mr. White's work: " Many millions of them have been brought to and born in America; most of them indeed have been confined to tillage, to their own homes, and their own society ; yet many of them have been so situated, that they might have availed themselves of the conversation of their masters; many have been brought up to the handicraft arts, and from that circumstance have always been associated with the whites. Some have been *liberally* educated," (with more truth it might be said *licentiously*,) " and all have lived in countries, where the arts and sciences are cultivated to a considerable degree, and have had samples of the best works from abroad. The

Indians *, with no advantages of this kind, will often carve figures on their pipes, not destitute of design and merit. They will crayon out an animal, a plant, or a country, so as to prove the existence of a germ in their minds, which only wants cultivation. They astonish you with strokes of the most sublime oratory, such as prove their reason and sentiment strong, their imagination glowing and elevated; but never yet could I find, that a black had ever uttered a thought above the level † of a plain narration, never see even an elementary trait of painting and sculpture." It is astonishing to find such assertions made by a man whose opportunities of information must have been extensive. In Africa, it is very customary for the natives to carve the outside of their calibashes, the handles of their spoons and weapons, in a variety of neat fancy patterns, some representing

* Dr. Smith, in his learned Essay on the Variety of Complexion in the Human Species, says, p. 81, " The exaggerated representations which we sometimes receive of the ingenuity and profound wisdom of savages (meaning the Americans) are the fruits of weak and ignorant surprise."

As it is not my wish to depreciate one kind of people in order to elevate another, I shall not give the picture of the North American Indian, drawn by Dr. Smith in the above mentioned work, (p. 84.) which does not indicate that degree of intellectual capacity which Mr. Jefferson attributes to them.—A very different account is also given of them by Dr. Douglas, in his Historical and Political History of the British Settlements in North America, vol. i. p. 153, where he says, speaking of the aboriginal inhabitants, " New negroes from Guinea generally exceed them much in constitution of body and mind."

† Can a man be eloquent in a language which he imperfectly understands?

human heads and faces, others depicting animals, &c. Among the native African boys, lately brought to England by the Sierra Leone company, are several whose genius for drawing is very remarkable, and whose copies are so accurate, that were it thought proper for them to pursue that line, not a doubt can be entertained of their rising to considerable eminence.

Mr. Imlay remarks, that Baron de Tott, speaking of the ignorance of the Turks, who are also slaves but whites, says, it was with difficulty that he could make them comprehend the simplest proposition in mathematics. Mr. Imlay further observes, " a black in New England has composed an ephemeris, which I have seen, and which men, conversant in the science of astronomy, declare, exhibits marks of acute reason and genius. ' Religion has produced a Phillis Wheatly ; but it could not produce a poet,' is another of Mr. Jefferson's dogmata. Phillis was brought from Africa to America, between seven and eight years of age ; and without any assistance from a school education, and before she was fifteen years old, wrote many of her poems. This information is attested by her then master, John Wheatly, dated Boston, Nov. 14, 1772." Mr. Imlay, in proof of his assertion, quotes a part of her beautiful Poem on Imagination ; but as it is too long, the following short extract from an Hymn to the Morning, may serve as a specimen of her poetical talents :

Aurora hail, and all the thousand dies,
Which deck thy progress through the vaulted skies:
The morn awakes, and wide extends her rays,
On every leaf the gentle zephyr plays ;
Harmonious lays the feather'd race resume,
Dart the bright eye, and shake the painted plume.

" As to the whites being more elegantly formed
(says Mr. Imlay) as asserted by Mr. Jefferson, I
must confess, that it has never appeared so to me.
On the contrary, I have often observed, in families
which have been remarkable for feeding their
blacks well, and treating them in other respects
with humanity, that their Negroes have been as
finely formed as any whites I ever saw.—Indeed,
my admiration has often been arrested, in examining their proportion, muscular strength, and ath-
letic powers."

Mr. Imlay concludes these remarks with a com-
pliment to Mr. Jefferson's candour and goodness
of heart, and adds an extract from his work, which
breathes such a spirit of truth, that I cannot refrain from inserting it. " The whole commerce
between master and slave is a perpetual exercise
of the most boisterous passions, the most unremit-
ting despotism on one part, and degrading sub-
missions on the other. Our children see this, and
learn to imitate it. The parent storms, the child
looks on, catches the lineaments of wrath, puts on
the same airs, gives a loose to his worst of passions,
and thus nursed, educated, and daily exercised in
tyranny, cannot but be stamped with odious peculiarities." After making several moral reflections

upon the subject of slavery, Mr. Jefferson finishes with these emphatical words : " Indeed, I tremble for my country, when I reflect that God is just : that his justice cannot sleep for ever: that, considering numbers, nature, and natural means only, a revolution of the wheel of fortune, an exchange of situation, is among possible events: that it may become probable by supernatural interference ! The Almighty has no attribute which can take side with us in such a contest."

SENSE OF FEELING.

The cuticle and rete mucosum are said to be thicker in the African than in the European, from which Mr. White draws this conclusion : " It is no wonder then, that Negroes have not that lively and delicate sense of touch that the whites have, since both the cuticle and rete mucosum are thicker in them.—In brutes, this sense is still duller than in Negroes." I doubt very much the accuracy of this observation, though I can adduce no direct proof of the contrary. We find in the European that the cuticle is *thicker*, and more deeply furrowed at the finger ends, the very seat of feeling, than it is in the face.

The African women have in general easy labours, but they do not " retire to the woods, bring forth alone, and return directly home." We have had in this country innumerable instances of unfortunate women bringing forth in private, and engaging immediately in fatiguing employments, in order to prevent suspicion, and preserve their character in society. Mr. White concludes the paragraph on parturition, with saying, that " women of colour have easier parturitions in general, than white Europeans; and that brutes have easier parturitions than the human species."

Having been present at a great number of labours among the Nova Scotian blacks at Sierra Leone, I can affirm, that they in every respect resemble those of women in the same situation of life in England ; and the observation may perhaps be extended to the Africans. I have met with instances in England, where the fœtus was expelled with more ease than I ever knew it to be at Sierra Leone. Instances of labour protracted to twenty-four hours and upwards, occurred frequently at Free Town ; and I knew some from the effects of which the patients suffered very severely. In every case, which came under my observation, there was the same relative proportion between the capacity of the pelvis and the head of the child as is found in England.

Mr. White next speaks of the DISEASES of black people. I have already said that I never met with an instance of tetanus in Africa. The insensibility of Negroes to pain, noticed by Dr. Mosely, if real, ought perhaps to be referred to that state of depression, and indifference to life, produced by West Indian slavery. No such fact is observable in Africa.

Mr. White proceeds to say, " European women, in hot countries, are very subject to floodings, and to the fluor albus. Negresses are almost exempt from both these complaints, but are very liable to obstructions of the *menses*." These assertions are far too general. Menorrhagia occurs sometimes, though rarely, among the natives; but I have met with several instances of it among the black settlers at Free Town. Obstructions of the menses rarely happen among the Africans or settlers, except as an effect of some tedious illness ; slaves in the West Indies, however, are very liable to them, in consequence of the debility occasioned by bad diet, depressing passions, &c. Fluor albus is a complaint to which we might expect a priori, that the natives of Africa would not be subject; it depends so much upon a peculiar mode of life, and is so much connected with certain affections of the mind, that it may be regarded as one of the attendants of civilization. It seldom appears among the black women at Free Town, but I have met, even among them, with some cases, as obstinate as any I have seen in England.

Dr. John Hunter, says, ' the cacabay is a negro name for a disease not known among Europeans or their descendants, as far as I could learn.' This assertion has been already noticed under the head of elephantiasis. The same author likewise mentions *dirt-eating*, as a disorder which is peculiar to Negroes, and frequently proves fatal to them. A species of this complaint, however, frequently occurs in England, in chlorosis, and in some cases of pregnancy.

I do not recollect having ever remarked, or hearing it remarked, that the African's manner of walking is very different from that of the European's."

Mr. White having thus attempted to prove that material differences exist in the organization and constitution of the human species, concludes by observing, that these differences " generally mark a regular gradation, from the white European down, through the human species, to the brute creation. From which it appears, that in those particulars wherein mankind excel brutes, the European excels the African."

" It remains yet to notice, that in those particular respects in which the brutes excel mankind, the African excels the European; these are chiefly the senses of *seeing*, *hearing*, and *smelling* ; the faculty of memory, and the power of *mastication*."

Mr. White has not favoured us with any instances of the superiority of the Africans in the above points, and I am persuaded that his remarks on this subject are perfectly unfounded. Mankind are so much inclined to pride themselves upon any point in which they may excel their fellow creatures, that there is no doubt, if the African possessed these advantages, that he would be disposed to boast of them ; but I never heard such a circumstance noticed, either by the Africans themselves, or by Europeans residing in Africa.

I observed in them, indeed, a superior quickness of discovering game in a forest; but this faculty is acquired by practice; for they by no means equal in this respect the acuteness of those American Indians who live solely upon the chace.

In England, persons not accustomed to hunting, will walk close to a hare upon her seat, without observing her, but she is instantly discovered by the eye of the sportsman. Mr. Browne, in his travels in Africa, says, that among the Negroes " there are few instances of myopes; and blindness is very uncommon." These remarks I believe to be just; I know no instances of blindness among them, except from accidents, the small-pox, or extreme old age. Whether they possess *strong eyes* or not, I cannot determine. In England, the black eye does not appear to possess the strongest sight.

Mr. White's objections to the Mosaic account of the creation, which are equally weak and futile with those of the infidel writers who have gone before him, are so fully and satisfactorily anticipated in Mr. Clarkson's " Essay on the Slavery and Commerce of the Human Species," (a work containing also much curious and accurate information respecting Africa and its inhabitants) that it is unnecessary to advert to them here.

APPENDIX N° IV.

THE following important and valuable remarks of Professor Blumenbach upon Negroes, are taken from " Voigts Magazin für das neueste aus der Physik *," &c. and afford ample testimony to the truth of what has been asserted respecting them.

" In the picture gallery at Pommersfeld, I saw four heads of Negroes by Vandyk†, of which, two in particular had so little of the projecting facial line, that they differed but in a small degree from the European countenance.

" At that time I had met with few opportunities of obtaining any knowledge of the form of the Negro head from nature ; and as it occurred to me that Mr. Camper had asserted, in a lecture delivered at the academy of painting in Amsterdam, that, " most of the great painters, and especially Rubens, Vandyk, and Jordaens, had instead of Negroes drawn only black coloured Europeans." I ascribed the agreeable forms of these Negro faces to this general error.

---

* Einige naturhistorische Bemerkungen bey Gelegenheit einer Scweizerreise. Vom Hrn. Prof. Blumenbach. 4. Bandes 3. Stück.

† See Verzeichn. der Schildereyen in der Gallerie des Hochgräflichen Schönbornischen Schlosses zu Pommersfelden.

" A few months afterwards, however, I had an opportunity of convincing myself, that there are real Negroes, whose lineaments agree with those of Europeans, and that the painting at Pommersfeld at least, might be an accurate representation of nature.

" Being about to visit Messrs. Treytorrens in Yverdun, one of whom had resided a long time in St. Domingo, as I entered the court yard of the house, I saw only a woman, standing with her back towards me, whose elegant form attracted my notice. But how much was I surprised, when on accosting her she turned round, to find a Negress, whose physiognomy perfectly corresponded with such a form, and, in my mind, completely justified the accuracy of the Negro portraits by Vandyk, which I had seen at Pommersfeld.

" Her face was such, that even the nose, and somewhat thicker lips, had nothing peculiar, certainly nothing unpleasant in their appearance; and had the same features occurred in a white skin, they would have excited very general admiration. To this were added, the most sprightly and cheerful vivacity, a sound judgment, and as I afterwards discovered, peculiar knowledge and skill in midwifery. The pretty Negress of Yverdun is widely celebrated as the best midwife in that part of Switzerland.

" I heard from her master (who had likewise in his service a Negro of a very elegant form) that she was a Creole from St. Domingo. Her parents

were from Congo, but not so black as the Senegambia Negroes.

" Since that time I have had an opportunity of
seeing and speaking with several Negroes, and
have also procured three skulls, and a number of
preparations from Negroes, for my collection. All
these circumstances, together with what I have
learned on the subject from books of travels, have
convinced me still more of the truth of the two following positions, viz.

" 1. Among Negroes, both with regard to colour, and still more, with respect to the facial
line, as many, if not more varieties, occur, as between the most perfect Negro and the other varieties of mankind.

" 2. Negroes with respect to their mental capa-
cities and talents, do not appear to be in the least
inferior to the other races of mankind.

" The very striking gradation observable in
three Negro skulls which I have before me, afford
an evident proof of the justness of the first position

" The first, which was brought from New York
by M. Michaelis, and which I have elsewhere
exactly described *, is distinguished by so projecting an upper jaw, that if all Negroes were the
same, we might be tempted to think that they
sprung from an Adam different from our own.

" The facial line of the third slopes so little, and
indeed is so different from the former, and has
so little exotic in its appearance, that if I had not
(through the goodness of M. Michaelis) dissected

* Osteologie, p. 87,

the entire head, exactly as it was separated from the fresh subject, I should have hesitated to call it the head of a genuine Negro.

" The second stands midway between the two others; and has in its whole form a great resemblance to the head of the Abyssinian Abbas Gregorius, of which I have a good plate, done by Heiss, in 1691, after Von Sand, and which shews the near affinity of the Abyssinians with the Negroes. It more nearly resembles the plain featured Negroes, according to European ideas of beauty, than those so finely formed as the Negress of Yverdun, or the innumerable fine negro faces to be met with which differ but little from those of Europeans.

" What I have here said respecting the resemblance of so many Negroes to Europeans, is only a confirmation of a fact which has been long known, and which has frequently been remarked by unprejudiced and attentive travellers, a few of whom I shall quote in proof of my assertion.

" Thus: Le Maire, in his Voyages aux Cap Verd, Senegal, et Gambie, p. 161, says, ' a l'exception de la noirceur, il y a des Negresses aussi bien faites que nos dames Europeanes.'

" Leguat in his Travels, vol ii. p. 136, observes, ' j'ai rencontré à Batavia plusieurs fort jolies Negresses. Un visage tout-a-fait formé à l'Européene.'

" Mr. Adanson's description of the Senegambia Negresses has already been noticed.

" Ulloa in the *Noticias Americanas,* vol. ii.

p. 92, says, ' among the Negroes some have thick protruded lips, a flat nose, deep seated eyes, which are commonly called getudos, and wool instead of hair. Others, whose colour is quite as black as the former, and whose features, especially the mouth, nose, and eyes, are similar to the whites, have long thick hair.

" The testimonies, and instances in proof of the second position above mentioned, namely, of the sound judgment, good natural capacity and genius of Negroes, are just as incontrovertible and numerous as those of the first.

" Their astonishing memory, their extensive commercial undertakings*, their acuteness in

---

* Barbot relates many curious particulars upon this subject in his excellent Description of the Coasts of North and South Guinea, in the 5th vol. of Churchill's Collection of Voyages.

Page 235, it is said, " The blacks are for the most part men of sense and wit enough ; of a sharp ready apprehension, and an excellent memory beyond what is easy to imagine ; for though they can neither read nor write, they are always regular in the greatest hurry of business and trade, and seldom in confusion."

A very accurate writer remarks, " it is astonishing with what facility the African brokers reckon up the exchange of European goods for slaves. One of these brokers has perhaps ten slaves to sell, and for each of these he demands ten different articles. He reduces them immediately by the head into bars, coppers, ounces, according to the part of the country in which he resides, and immediately strikes the balance."—" On those parts of the coast, which are the greatest markets for slaves, many Africans reside, who act as interpreters to the ships. These, by great industry and perseverance, have made themselves masters of two or three of the languages of the country, and of the language of those Europeans with whom they are most connected in trade."—" Several of the African traders or great men, are not unacquainted with letters. This is particularly the case at Bonny and Calibar, where they not only speak the English language with fluency, but *write* it. These traders send letters repeatedly to the merchants here, trade, particularly with gold dust, in which the most experienced European traders cannot always be sufficiently upon their guard, are circumstances too well known to require repetition.

" The singular facility with which slaves learn all kinds of fine hand-work, is likewise well known.

" The same may be said of their musical talents *; we have had instances of Negroes who performed upon the violin in so masterly a manner, and gained so much money by it, as to be enabled to pay a large sum to purchase their freedom †.

" Of the poetical genius of Negroes we have well known instances in both sexes.

" Mons. Von Haller mentions a Negress who was a poetess.

" A specimen of the Latin poems of the Negro, Francis Williams, an excellent schoolmaster, are contained in the History of Jamaica.

" The Negro, Ignatius Sancho, has lately introduced himself to general notice by his interesting letters.

stating the situation of the markets, the goods which they would wish to be sent out to them the next voyage, the number of slaves which they expect to receive by that time, and such other particulars as might be expected from one merchant to another."— *On the Slavery and Commerce of the Human Species*, p. 125.

* This is contrary to the opinion of Mr. Bryan Edwards; but it is maintained by others equally eminent. Mr. Clarkson observes, " they play upon a variety of instruments, without any other assistance than their own ingenuity. They have also tunes of their own composition. Some of these have been imported among us, are now in use, and are admired for their sprightliness and ease, though the ungenerous and prejudiced importer has concealed their original." *On the Slavery and Commerce of the Human Species*.

† Hrn. Urlspergers Americanish Ackerwerk Gottes, S. 311.

" To the above instances may be added two others, to shew the genius and talents of our black brethren for scientific acquirements.

" It is well known that the protestant minister James John Eliza Capitein was a Negro, and a learned man, and a good orator. I have his portrait in an excellent plate by Tanjé, after P. Van Dyk.

" Professor Hollman, when at Wittenberg, conferred the degree of Doctor of Philosophy upon a Negro who had greatly distinguished himself, and who afterwards went to Berlin as a privy counsellor. (Konigl. Preuss. Hofrath.) I have in my possession two of his dissertations, one of which in particular contains much unexpected and well digested erudition, drawn from the best physiological works of that time. Its title is Diss. Inaug. philosophica de humanæ Mentis απαθεια, s. Sensionis ac Facultatis in Mente humana Absentia, & earum in Corpore nostro organico ac vivo Præsentia, quam Præs. D. Mart. Goth. Loeschero publice defendit auctor Ant. Guil. Amo Guinea—Afer, Phil. & A. A. L. L. Mag. & J. V. C. Wittebergæ, 1734, m. Apr.

" The title of the other is Disp. Philosophica continens Ideam distinctam eorum quæ competunt vel Menti vel Corpori nostro vivo & organico, quam Præside M. Ant. Guil. Amo Guinea—Afro d. 29 Maii 1734, defendit Io. Theodos. Meiner Rochliz Misnic. Philos. & J. V. Cultor.

" In an account of the life of Amo, which on this occasion was printed in the name of the academic council, it is said among other particulars respecting his talents: " Honorem meritis ingenii partum, insigni probitatis, industriæ, eruditionis, quam publicis privatisque exercitationibus declaravit, laude auxit.——Compluribus philosophiam domi tradidit, excusissimam veterum, quam novorum, placitis; optima quæquæselegit, selecta enucleate, ac dilucide interpretatus est."

" The president, at the public defence of the first dissertation, says expressly to Amo in the following congratulatory speech: " Tuum potissimum eminet ingenium felicissimum——utpote qui istius felicitatem atque præstantiam, eruditionis ac doctrinæ soliditatem ac elegantiam multis speciminibus hactenus in nostra etiam academia magno cum applausu omnibus bonis, & in præsenti dissertatione egregie comprobasti. Reddo tibi illam proprio marte eleganter ac erudite elaboratam, integram adhuc & plane immutatam, ut vis ingenii tui eo magis exinde elucescat."——

" Boerhaave and De Haen have given the most flattering testimonies of the uncommon progress of several negroes in the practice of medicine, and the science and skill of the midwife of Yverdun are, as has been already said, universally celebrated in that neighbourhood.

" Finally, the academy of sciences at Paris includes amongst its correspondents a Negro, Monsr. Lislet, in the Isle of France, who excels in the accuracy of his meteorological observations.

" From the instances already adduced, it is to

be hoped that my assertion will be justified respecting the equality of the Negroes to us other
children of Adam.

"On the other hand, I should think many considerable provinces of Europe might be named,
from which it would be difficult to produce a vir-
tuoso, a poet, a philosopher, and correspondent of
the Paris Academy."—

INDEX

SECOND VOLUME.

———

A

Page

ABOMA snake, described by Capt. Stedman 179
Abortion, artificial, seldom attempted in Africa............................. 215
Abscess of the liver, a rare occurrence 120
Africans, their notions of medicine blended with magic...................... 10
————— suppose the stomach the chief seat of disease ... . ib.
————— not exempt from remittent fever 14
————— hasten the approach of old age by intemperance 115
————— mental faculties of the, noticed 264
————— boys brought to England by the Sierra Leone Company 268
Agues, rarely observed among the Bulloms and Timmanees 21
————— more frequent among the Foolas .... ib.
————— how treated by the natives .... ib.
Ague cakes, rarely occur among the Africans 22
————————— very frequent among resident Europeans..................... ib.
————————— falsely attributed to the use of the Peruvian bark 23
Amo, a learned Negro, Doctor of Philosophy. 281
Anasarca, occurring in children 222
Anorexia, or loss of appetite, how treated 124
Ants, black, incredible swarms of 176
Aphrodisiacs, in great request among the Mahommedans 114
Apothecary, the art of the, noticed in Scripture 6
Apthous, ulcers of the mouth, how treated 41
Ardor urinæ, in gonorrhœa, how relieved 35
Aristotle, his opinion respecting the tide....................................... 11
Arm of the negro not longer than in Europeans 256
Arsenic used by the Hindoos in elephantiasis 60
Atkins describes the credulity of a British governor 11

INDEX.

B

Page

Bark, African, mistaken for a species of rondeletia 243
——————— efficacious in fevery sore throat, dysentery, &c.... .....45, 247
——————— cases of its efficacy .... 247, & seq.
—— Peruvian, false opinions respecting its use 23
Belly *sick*, fever often so termed by the Africans 13
—— pendulous, how prevented 264
Blafard, Chacrelas, or white negro, described................................ 172
Bleeding from an artery or vein unknown to the Africans 20
———— said to have been practised by the Egyptians .... ib.
Blindness, night, occasionally occurs in Africa............................ 128
——————— how remedied, according to Pliny .... ib.
Blood, flux of, from wounds, how restrained 200
Blumenbach, Professor, his remarks on negroes. Appendix. No. IV. 275
Boys, African, brought over by the Sierra Leone Company 268
Breasts, *milk*, medical treatment of 217
—— pendulous, how occasioned............................... 264
Bulloms, their opinion respecting death 10
Burns and scalds, applications made to............... 193

C

Cachexia Africana described 225
Calculous complaints not frequent on the coast of Africa 35
——————— more common in the desert .... ib.
Calypso, the, transport, refitted at Sierra Leone 16
Capitein, J. J. E. a learned negro.. 281
Capsicum or red pepper, used in the cure of dysentery.................... 44
Catamenia, curious opinions concerning the 205
Cautery, actual, employed by the natives of Fezzan 119
——————— to restrain hæmorrhage from wounds 202
Cephalics, a very numerous class of African remedies 17
Chigoes, a frequent complaint in the West Indies 107
—— mode of extracting, described by Ligon 108
Child birth, circumstances respecting 209
Children, negro, a vulgar error respecting 116
—— how carried by their mothers 221
—— diseases and management of 219
—— deformed, rarely seen 222
—— how long suckled........................... 218
—— subject to various eruptions 222
—— a species of anasarca................................. ib.
Chin of the negro, a supposed peculiarity of 256

INDEX.

	Page
Circumcision, various particulars respecting	229
Climate, effects of, on the African constitution	260
Cochin leg, described by Dr. Clark	114
Cold and moisture, effects of, on the human body	261
Cholic pains of the bowels, not unfrequent	46
————— remedies for, very numerous	47
Consumption, seldom idiopathic	120
————— very frequent among the Spanish Indians	ib.
————— how treated by the Africans	121
Convalescents, treatment of	25
Corpulency sometimes occurs as a disease	131
Cough, usual mode of treatment of	121
Coup de soleil, a species of apoplexy	38
————— fatal effects of, in China	39
Croup, a case of, occurring at Free Town	130
Cupping, mode of performing in Africa	20
Customs not easily changed in hot climates	9

D

Diseases of the African, compared with those of the Europeans	271
————— general, to which both sexes are liable	13
————— of women	205
————— of children	219
Dirt eating, dreadful effects of	225
Dondo or white negro, described	172
Dracunculus, occurs in many parts of Africa	82
————— most frequent on the Gold Coast	83
————— considered by some authors as an epidemic	85
————— described by Mr. Bruce	87, 92
————— mode of cure generally practised	95
————— frequently exists in the body unsuspected	98
————— cases of	100, & seq.
Druids, priests and physicians of the Gauls and Britons	8
Duration of the life of the African shortened by intemperance	262
Dysentery, dreadful effects of, in slave vessels	42
————— most frequent on the Gold Coast	44
————— how treated there	45

E

Ear, pains of, how treated by the Africans	42
Egypt, termed by Homer the land of physicians	7
Elephantiasis, why so called	50
————— various names applied to it by authors	ib.
————— imported from Egypt into Italy	51

INDEX.

Page

Elephantiasis, very frequent during the ninth century in Europe............ 52
——————- described as it occurs in South America 53
——————- case of, described in a Foola .... ib.
——————- divided into different species by the Foolas 57
——————- supposed to be contagious 53
——————- cured in the East Indies by means of arsenic 60
Enema, mode of administering 45
Enlargement of the scrotum to an immense size 110
——————— of the scrotum, case of, in a fine young man 111
——————— of the legs frequent on the Gold Coast 113
Epilepsy, sometimes occurs in Africa 45
——————- names applied to it by the natives............................... 26
Eunuchs not subject to elephantiasis... 67
Euphorbia tithymaloides recommended in syphilis 32
European credulity, an instance of 11
Europeans, when said to be *seasoned*............ 14
Exomphalos, frequent in African children 223
External senses of the African, compared with those of the European 273
Eyes, diseases of, not frequent in Africa................................. ... 127
—— inflammation of the, how treated 129

F

Feeling, sense of, less acute in the African than European 270
Fever, frequent among Europeans in Africa 13
——- no name for, in the African languages............................... ib.
——- malignant, of the West Indies, supposed to have been introduced
    from Africa............................. 15
—— of Sierra Leone, resembles that of Bulam 16
Fezzan, diseases of, how treated by the natives 118
Fractured limbs, usual mode of treatment............................ 203
Framboesia, or yaws, described 139
——————— improperly divided into species 145
——————— case of an European affected with............................. 146
——————— mistaken for the venereal disease 148
——————— said to be communicable to animals 153
——————— well described by Dr. Schilling 159
——————— introduced by inoculation, on the Gold Coast.................. 156
Frogs frequently found in trees.. 181

G

Glands of the neck tumefied... .... 30, 223
Gonorrhœa, frequent among the Africans....................................... 34
——————- mode of treatment adopted .... ib.
Gout, a disease unknown in Africa 114

INDEX.

                                                                      Page

Gradation, regular, in man, remarks on the.................................. 254
Guinea worm described 82
————- most frequent on the Gold Coast 84
————- caused by drinking bad water 88
————- Mr. Bruce's description of the 92
Gypsies, or fortune-tellers, among the antients.............................. 6

H

Hæmoptysis, a case of, how treated............................... 125
Hæmorrhage from wounds, how restrained 200
Hands and feet of the negroes, remarks on the 256
Hankey, the, transport had no communication with Sierra Leone 16
Head-ach in fever, treatment of, by the Africans 17
————- how treated by the Mongearts 21
———— sick, often applied to fever....................................... 13
Hernia humoralis, not an unfrequent disease 36
Herniæ, not common among the Africans 37
————- improperly attributed to the use of oil .... ib.
————- confounded with swelled testicle 38
Herpes, or ringworm, how treated by the natives 163
Hydrocele, frequent among the Moors... 36
Hysteria, an uncommon disease in Africa 205

I

Idiotism, rarely occurs as an idiopathic disease 25
Imlay, Mr. his refutation of Mr. Jefferson's remarks........................ 265
Indian remedies for the venereal disease.. 33
————- their efficacy called in question .... ib.
Indians, the priests of the, are physicians and conjurors....................... 8
Indigestion, how treated 124
Infants, treatment of 214
Injection for the cure of gonorrhœa 35
Inoculation of the small pox unknown at Sierra Leone 135
————- practised in some parts of the country .... ib.
————- unsuccessful among black people in cold countries 136
———— for the yaws, used on the Gold Coast 156
Intermittents rarely occur among the natives 21
————- how treated in general........ .... ib.
————- uncommon among slaves in the West Indies 22
————- frequent among the Nova Scotian Settlers .... ib.
Itch, or kra-kra, very common among the Africans 164

J

Jefferson, Mr. his remarks on the mental faculties of the African......... 265

INDEX.

K

                                                                      Page
Kra-kra, or itch, various names for... 164
———- remedies used for the cure of... 165

L

Laanda, a kind of phagædenic ulcer, resembling lues 33
Labours of the women, generally easy........., ... 209
———- inference drawn from thence, by Mr. White..................... ... 270
Leather dyed red by a vegetable infusion............ 19
Lethargy, or *sleepy sickness*, frequent in Africa... 29
——— generally proves fatal 30
Leucæthiops, or white negro, opinions of authors respecting 166
———— solitary instances only of this disease..................... ..... ib.
——— compared with the Cretins of the lower Vallais 171
Lime bush, the leaves of the, used in head-ache 18
——— much celebrated for its virtues by the antients 123
——— juice, used in the cure of dysentery 44
Lislet, Monsr. a negro, and accurate meteorologist 282
Lobelia, recommended in the cure of syphilis............................. 33
———- its efficacy doubted by Dr. Rush .... ib.
Longevity, a well authenticated instance of, in an African................. 114
——— fewer instances of longevity among negroes, than Europeans 262
Lumbago, how cured by the Africans 118

M

Maladie du pays, nostalgia, acts powerfully on the African 174
Mal d'Estomac, Cachexia Africana, described 225
Mal rouge of Cayenna, a species of elephantiasis 53
Man, the supposed regular gradation in 254
Mania, rarely occurs in Africa 25
Measles, a rare occurrence 137
———- mode of treatment of .... ib.
Medical remedies, discovery of, borrowed from animals..................... 5
Medicine, progress of, slow in the beginning 4
——— practised by the rudest nations .... ib.
——— origin of, described by Seneca .... ib.
———— described by Quintilian 5
——— and religion originally united 6
——— practice of, in high repute among the antients 7
——— union of, with magic in the early ages 8
——— in Africa, not in an improving state................................. 9
Medicines, not supposed to be influenced by the phases of the moon...... 10

INDEX.

Page

Mercury, its speedy effects on the mouth 23
Milk breasts, how treated................. 217
Miscarriages, superstitious notions respecting 216
———————- the disposition to, how treated .... ib.
Mongearts, an African nation, their cure for head-ach 21
Moisture, combined with cold and heat, effects of........................ 261

N

Nauclea sambucina, used for the cure of dysentery 45
Navel, prodigiously enlarged 224
Negroes, new, not exempt from yellow fever................................ 15
———————- in the West Indies rarely affected with ague 22
———————- capable of resisting cold as well as Europeans 262
———————- skeleton of the, compared with the European 254
———————- white, supposed to form a distinct nation........................ .. 166
———————————— instances of the, described 167
———————————— improperly compared with Cretinism 171
New South Wales, height of the thermometer there 261
Nostalgia, not peculiar to Switzerland... 174
Nova Scotian Settlers at Free Town liable to agues....... 22
Nyctalopia, or night blindness, instances of 128

O

Obia men in the West Indies, like the agyrtæ of the antients.............. 7
Oedema of the lower extremities not unfrequent 24
————————————————— how treated by the natives .... ib.
Ophthalmia, remedies employed in 129
Otaheite, at, the office of physician and priest united 9

P

Pastinaca marina, case of a man stung by............................. 191
Pectoral complaints, various remedies for 122
Pemphigus, how treated by the natives... 137
Phases of the moon, not attended to in collecting simples.................... 11
Philips, his humane description of a slave ship 42
Phips, General, his superstition noticed by Atkins 11
Phlegmone testis, not an unfrequent occurrence, and why................... 36
Physicians mentioned by the sacred writers 6
Piso, his opinion respecting the tide... 11
Placenta, expulsion of the, how promoted 212
Pleurisy, not a common disease in Africa 119
Pliny, his account of the origin of medicine 5
Poison, how expelled from the stomach 124
——— of snakes, not hurtful in the stomach 188

INDEX.

	Page
Poison *fish*, curious effects of the	173
Polysarcia, or corpulency, occurs as a disease	131
Prolapsus ani, how treated	224
Psylli, art of the, unknown on the coast of Africa	185
———– account of the, in Egypt	186
Puberty, mistake concerning the period of	262
Purgative medicine, a violent	125
——————— recommended in belly-ach	ib.

Q

Quintilian, his description of the origin of medicine	5

R

Religion in the early ages united with medicine	6
Rheumatism, not uncommon in Africa	116
——————— mode of cure adopted by the natives	117
Rice supposed to be prejudicial to the eyes	127
Ricinus, the leaves of, applied in head-ach	18
————————— in œdematous swellings	24
Rickets, a rare disease in Africa	224
Rum, virtues attributed to it by the Foolas	27
Ruptures, Africans not very subject to	37
Rush, Dr. shews the difficulty of attaining a knowledge of the Indian art of medicine	2

S

Sailors become sooner infirm than any other classes of men	263
Salivation excited by vegetables as a cure for syphilis	33
Sancho Ignatius, a negro of good abilities	280
Sarcoma scrotale, a frequent disease in Africa	110
——————— prevails most in certain districts	ib.
——————— a frequent complaint in Galam	112
Scalds, how treated by the Africans	193
Scorpion, bite of, attended with acute pain	188
——————— how treated by the natives	189
——————— case of, in a black woman	190
Scrophula sometimes met with in Africa	120
Scurvy unknown in Africa	41
Scurvy suspected to occur frequently in slave ships	42
Seasoning, signification of the term	14
Sibbens, or sivvens, compared with yaws	154
Skeleton of the negro compared with the European	254
Skin, diseases of the, most common in Africa	163
——— mottled appearance of the	173

INDEX.

	Page
Sleepy sickness, its symptoms and treatment	29
Small pox, supposed to originate in Africa	132
———— its last appearance on the Windward coast	133
———— how treated by the natives	134
———— fatality of, in North America	136
Snakes, flesh of, not used medicinally by the Africans.................	66
———— several poisonous kinds of	177
———— of immense size called tennay	179
———— contest between a, and a frog........................	181
———— bites of, how treated by the Africans	182
———————— supposed antidotes for	184
———— much dreaded by the natives	185
———— fascinated by the inhabitants of Sennaar........	186
Spitting of blood, how treated by the Africans.................	125
Sting ray, case of a man bitten by	191
Suckling of children, how long continued...................	218
Sumatrans pretend to cure syphilis without mercury	32
Sun stroke, a rare occurrence in Africa	38
————- seldom affects Europeans there...........	39
————- too frequently the effect of strong liquors	ib.
————- treatment of	40
Surgeons of slave vessels, their degraded situation exposed.............	43

T

Tennay, a snake of prodigious size	179
Tetters, or ring worm, medical treatment of....................	163
Theft, how punished among the Foolas	201
Thirst in fevers, how remedied	16
Throat, sore, medical treatment of..............................	131
Tide, supposed to influence departing life	11
Tinea capitis, treatment of	222
Toma, or poison tree, used in œdematous swellings	25
Tooth-ach, not unfrequent in Africa	40
———————— remedies for	ib.
Trismus nascentium, does not affect the African children	220
———————————— occurs frequently in the West Indies	221
Twins, curious opinion of the Foolas concerning	204

U

Ulcers, a numerous class of diseases	193
———— how dressed by the Africans	194
———— various remedies for	195
———— scrophulous, a case of...........................	196

INDEX.

V

	Page
Van Helmont, his opinion respecting death	10
Vena medinensis, or guinea worm	82
——————— called also pharoum, or Pharaoh's worm	87
——————— mode of extracting it	95
Venereal disease, pretended to be cured without mercury	32
——————— generally introduced by Europeans	ib.
Vermifuge remedies, a list of	28
Vomiting in fevers, how remedied by the natives	17

W

Wheatly, Phillis, an African poetess	268
White, Mr. remarks on his work on the gradation in man	25
Williams, Francis, a negro schoolmaster	280
Women, diseases peculiar to	205
Worms considered as a cause of disease	26
——— tape, frequent among the Foolas	ib.
——— how supposed to be produced	28
——— various remedies for	ib.
Wounds, the general treatment of	200

Y

Yaws, names applied to the disease by the Africans	139
——— symptoms of, described	140
——— how communicated	141
——— Dr. Mosely's opinion concerning, controverted	143
——— master, or mother, what	144
——— case of an European affected with	146
——— confounded by writers with the venereal disease	148
——— said to be communicable to animals	153
——— supposed to be a species of leprosy	154
——— a disease in Scotland so called	ib.
——— inoculation, for the, on the Gold Coast	156
——— how treated by the natives	157
Yellow billed sprat, fatal effects of the, when eaten	173

THE END.

ERRATA IN THE SECOND VOLUME.

Page 36, line 29, for *Ronnetookee* read *Konnetookee.*
38, — 3, for *Rookrakoonee* read *Kookrakoonee*
43, — 20, after *quantity* insert ''
43, — 29, before *the master* insert "
44, last line, for *fournier* read *fournir.*
51, line 24, for *lenticul* read *lenticula.*
52, — 17, after *imported* insert *or.*
89, — 19, for *Moors* read *Boors.*
112, — 30, after *food* add *as a condiment.*
125, — 4, for *cureas* read *curcas.*
133, — 25, for *Rocundy* read *Kocundy.*
135, *Note,* for *chemier* read *chenier.*
158, line 5, dele *in*
165, — 20, after *Tamba* insert a comma.
168, bottom, for *twink* read *twinkling.*
174, line 4, for *Epidermiss* read *Epidermis.*
177, — 11, for *Rangree* read *Kangree.*
195, — 27, after *Pongia* insert a comma.

.

For EU product safety concerns, contact us at Calle de José Abascal, 56–1°,
28003 Madrid, Spain or eugpsr@cambridge.org.

www.ingramcontent.com/pod-product-compliance
Ingram Content Group UK Ltd.
Pitfield, Milton Keynes, MK11 3LW, UK
UKHW040617240426
470322UK00010B/167